Autism:
Handle with Care!

Understanding and Managing the Behaviour of Children and Adults with Autism

Gail Gillingham

Tacit Publishing Inc., Edmonton, Alberta, Canada

Fourth Edition, Printed 08/01

Tacit Publishing Inc.
8744 - 81 Avenue,
Edmonton, Alberta, T6C 0W6
Canada

Telephone: 780-466-2445 Fax: 780-463-6433
E-mail: tacit@telusplanet.net

ISBN #09687863-0-8

To contact the author, Gail Gillingham, write to

Box 11245, Main Post Office
Edmonton, Alberta, T5J 3K5
Canada

Table of Contents

This book is dedicated to

Arthur, David and James,

who first taught me to care,

and to Kurt,

whose untimely death reminded me

that there is no time to waste.

Acknowledgments

In 1988, I was hired as a supervisor for a group home and stepped into a world I did not even know existed: the world of autism. Since that time I have come to know a very special group of people who live all over the world, and who affect me in ways no one else ever has. I love you.

This book is written for all of you: men, women, teenagers and children with autism. I can only hope that I have conveyed the message wisely and appropriately so that it makes a difference in your lives. Celebrate your unique abilities; feel free to be yourselves.

This book is also for all the parents, teachers, professionals and caregivers who have been so frustrated by the syndrome of autism. I understand how it feels to desperately want to help while at the same time being baffled by inappropriate and bizarre behaviours. I have been there through twenty-four hour care and have longed for any response -- anything that would make the hours seem worthwhile. Most of all, I have been involved with change. I have reached individuals as I discovered the reasons behind their behaviours. This is the message of hope I want to share with you.

I do not claim any ownership of this message, for it is the message of the people who actually have autism. I am totally indebted to their words on this topic and base everything I do and say on their experiences. I feel privileged to have had the time and opportunity to tie these words together and develop a whole picture, which hopefully is understandable to everyone who reads this book. If we heed these words, we will have the ability to improve the lives of all those who have autism.

Throughout the years I have taken carrying out research and writing this book, many people have been beside me in many different ways. I want all of you to know that I have appreciated you deeply. A heartfelt declaration of gratitude goes out to:

· First, and foremost, the many individuals with autism who are speaking out on how it feels to have autism. Special thanks to Temple Grandin, Darren White, Steven Stanton, Dietmar Zoller, David Eastham, Therese Marie Ronan, Sean Barron, Simon Morphett, Georgiana Manly, Donna Williams, Jeffrey Powell, Thomas McKean, Sara Miller, Birger Sellin, Ian Whetherbee, Dan Treacy, Wally Wojtowicz, Jr., Sue Rubin and Sharisa Kochmeister. Without you, this book would not have been possible.

· Margaret of Great Britain, who first introduced me to the role of endorphins in autism and who so willingly shared all her research in this area. I would also like to thank her for sharing my first paper, ***Listen to the Children***, with her many contacts, and for her wonderful hospitality while I was in England.

· The many parents from across the world who responded to my first article, ***Listen to the Children***: especially Liv Evans and Enid Stanton, whose letters continue to keep me going.

· The many parents, who have trusted me with their children and with their stories. Special thanks to John Manning, whose early morning phone calls from Australia, and Joan Latimer, whose letters and updates from Alberta, reminded me that I did have a job to do during 1992 when it would have been so easy to give up. Both had early rough copies of this book, and tested this method of care on their children; John as a father and Joan as a teacher.

· Dr. Vince Salvo at the Grande Prairie Regional College who was willing to spend the time to listen to my theory in the beginning and support it by introducing it to a first year class in sociology as a possible example of the attribution theory.

· Dr. James Park of the Royal Alexandra Hospital in Edmonton, who also listened and suggested that autism may well be the extreme on the extroverted/introverted scales and that I should take into consideration the work of Hans Eysenck.

· Dr. Paul Shattock and Gillian Lowden of the Autism Research Unit at the University of Sunderland in Sunderland, Great Britain for all their support. Their ***Titles in Autism*** has been an invaluable tool for my research. Their interest and enthusiasm continue with the development of a study to test this hypothesis by measuring the response levels of many individuals with autism.

· The many professionals who wrote letters of support and interest in my research; especially Dr. Margaret Creedon, Dr. Margaret Bauman, Dr. Karl Reichelt, Dr. William Condon, Dr. Peter Milner, Dr. Hans Eysenck, Barbara Hopkins, and Laura Cesaroni. Your words of encouragement have kept me on track.

· Dorothy Berg at the Hythe Public Library, who was so instrumental in my use of the interlibrary loan system and trusted me enough to order all the articles I requested, even if she was not sure those words existed.

· The various people at the University of Calgary Press who so patiently answered my letters and phone calls, and who did not forget me as the months flew by. Special thanks to Linda Cameron for her initial support and to John King for his words of advice.

· My four wonderful sons, Michael, Darryl, Timothy, and Gregory, as well as the students at the Western Arctic Leadership Program, who willingly put up with a "mother" who was so often lost in the world of autism. Your love and support is greatly appreciated.

· My parents, who provided me with a loving, stable home and who taught me so much, especially to care for others. Thanks for always being available, no matter what, and showing a real interest in whatever I was doing, even when you did not always understand. Thanks also to my sisters and brother and their families for their constant support.

· My terrific daughter-in-law, Lynne, whose enthusiasm and pride in my accomplishments boosts my spirits whenever we are in contact.

· Joshua and Matthew who have provided me with a new title -- grandmother -- and who supply the opportunity to watch the wonder of human growth all over again. Your hugs and kisses rebuild my spirit.

· And most of all to Clayton, who was there for me when my whole world fell apart, and who, through his love, encouragement, and support, gave me the freedom to concentrate all my energies on finishing this work.

Thanks so much to all of you.

Introduction

A Confusing Picture

Daniel is a three-year old child, taken to the Glenrose Hospital for tests. Garbage can lids are dropped directly behind him in order to check his hearing. He shows absolutely no response.

Is he deaf?

"No" says his mother, "he can't be. This is the same child who will run from one end of the house to the other, if he hears me unwrapping the cellophane off a piece of candy."

One Sunday afternoon, I supervise a group of autistic young men who have the job of cleaning up the yard, after a garden party. One of the crew, Sean, has been tested and is diagnosed legally blind. He is part of the group and all are expected to do their share. The staff believe that he is able to see more than his tests indicate. As we work together, I notice that the pieces of garbage Sean picks up are smaller than my little fingernail. If blind, how is he able to find these tiny scraps?

As a worker in the field of autism, these contradictions in autistic behaviour fascinate me. The apparent on again/off again ability for those who have autism to hear or not to hear, to see or not to see and so on, may well play an important part in the development of each individual. Just how this fits into the picture of autism, and how important its role may be, seems well worth investigating.

Breaking Through

Autism is the most difficult of developmental disorders with which to work. There is no known cause. There is no cure. Due to a lack of verbal ability on the part of most individuals with autism, we cannot ask them what is wrong. Their behaviour often seems bizarre and unpredictable. Caring for the autistic population often tends to feel like a thankless chore as clients show little or no response. Hours and hours of caretaker time are spent trying to reach those who have autism, to change their behaviours and make them normal and socially acceptable -- often to no avail.

This book concentrates on hope for people with autism through acceptance and understanding. This book is also about change, drastic change, and not only on the part of the autistic individual. Change must also occur within each caregiver. Beliefs and attitudes carried all our lives must be broken and discarded. Common assumptions held throughout society must be ignored. It is not an easy task, but it is imperative we make these changes in order to reach those who have autism.

Each of us fully believes that what we see, hear, and experience in this world is the same as any other person. For some reason, it is acceptable that there may be people who cannot see, hear or feel as much as we do. We give them labels of blind, deaf or mute and create ways and tools to normalize their situation as much as possible. On the other hand, it seems to be impossible for us to believe that someone could be on the other end of the scale: that someone is able to hear, see, or feel *more* than you or me.

In the past, having lived with a husband, who was colour blind, I was constantly surprised when reminded that the world we shared looked totally different to him than it did to me. Although I knew about his colour blindness for twenty-four years, I still found myself amazed when he picked the wrong shirt if I asked him to get my red one, or thought that a certain car belonged to a friend of ours when it, obviously, was a different colour. However, acceptance of this difference was not too difficult. After all, it had a label. He had the defect. There was a definite reason for his behaviour.

Experiences on the upper end of a sensory scale are more difficult to deal with. In a town in New Mexico, families are feuding; marriages are breaking up; and people are declaring friends, neighbours, and loved ones crazy.[1] These people are distracted, irritated, and having trouble with their sense of balance. Why? According to them a sound is emanating from the ground, a low throbbing sound that is driving them to distraction. The rest of the citizens have no sympathy for those who are suffering. They do not hear any sound. Therefore, those who claim to hear it obviously do not know what they are talking about.

When scientists visited this New Mexico town to measure the offending noise, they discovered that it actually exists. It oscillates between seventeen and twenty hertz. It is audible only to people with very acute hearing. The source of the sound is still a mystery and many continue to argue its existence. For these people, the logic is simple: if you can't hear the sound, it is just not there.

This book will take a close look at a group of people who hear sounds that we cannot hear, who see better than any of us can imagine, and whose sense of touch is so strong they cannot endure physical contact. Like the citizens of the New Mexico community, this group of people has been labelled. They are called crazy, schizophrenic, developmentally delayed, mentally retarded, and autistic. Each day of their lives, they not only have to deal with stimuli which we do not even know exists, but they have to cope with overwhelming stimulation from an environment that is quite normal and acceptable to us.

At present, many in the scientific world assume that all people have the same natural limits imposed on their sensory systems. Nature supposedly limits the amount of stimuli coming in and prevents brains from becoming overloaded with information.[2] This assumption has led to the establishment of a normal range of feeling, a range within which people are tested to see whether or not they are disabled. Since this assumption is so firmly entrenched in a great deal of our scientific thinking, rarely does anyone take the time to test for sensitivity above the normal range. If such a super sensitivity is a possibility, the next question is rather logical. What would be the short and long term effects on the development of a supersensitive person?

This book is a collection of the words of actual people who are affected by autism and of parents and caregivers who have taken note of the sensory responses of the people with whom they work. In taking the words of those with autism to heart, one comes to the obvious conclusion that a maximum range of sensitivity for all people is indeed not true. There are people who see, hear, smell, and feel with a sensitivity that is far above the normal range. The long-term result on their development is the autistic lifestyle. By ignoring this normal range assumption of sensory response and moving on, parents and caregivers can finally reach autistic individuals on their own level.

Throughout this book, people who have described how it feels to be autistic are mentioned by first and last name. These include Temple Grandin, Darren White, Steven Stanton, Dietmar Zoller, David Eastham, Therese Marie Ronan, Sean Barron, Simon Morphett, Georgiana Manly, Donna Williams, Jeffrey Powell, Thomas McKean, Wally Wojtowicz, Birger Sellin, Ian Whetherbee, Sharisa Kochmeister, Dan Treacy, Sue Rubin and Sara Miller. Without them, this book would not have been possible.

The use of personal accounts may lead readers to believe that this method of care is only applicable for people with autism who are high functioning. This is not correct. The stories included throughout this book, using only first names, are true stories that I have experienced myself, or which others have shared with me. Many of the people named in these stories are considered as very low functioning. Changes in their lives have been brought about by the methods described in this book, and by the realization by caregivers that many of the problems in the lives of people with autism are caused by their reactions to sensory stimulation. Low-functioning individuals with autism have higher levels of sensory response than those who are high functioning. Thus, they have greater need to protect themselves from the environment and spend most of their lives isolated in a world of their own.

We will not offer a cure. Instead, we provide hope by giving those who have autism an understanding hand through accepting their actual feelings and experiences. Then we go on to teach them how to cope with the reality of their situation and with the environments in which they live. By learning to cope, they can indeed have a chance to take their own rightful place as self-sufficient people in our society.

Super sensitivity to stimulation is not something new in the field of autism. It was first written about in 1949 by Bergman and Escolona[3] and has appeared in the scientific literature every now and then since. Many people tell me that they have always known that many individuals with autism are supersensitive. However, this is not being taught in our universities. It is not the focus of most scientific studies. It is not the accepted reality of the professional world. It is not what parents are being told. And it is not the message being delivered by autism societies around the world. Even when super sensitivity is recognized, the implications on the behaviour of the person with autism, are rarely recognized nor is the problem dealt with in any way. Therefore, I felt the need to write this book.

1 M. Haederle & P. Lambert, "Hmmmmmmmmmmmm...?" *People Weekly* (Vol. 38:12, 1992) pp. 61-62.

2 J. D. Barrow, *Theories of Everything: The Quest for the Ultimate Experience.* (Oxford, Clarendon Press, 1991) p. 11.

3 P. Bergman and S. Escalona, "Unusual sensitivities in very young children," *Psychoanalytic Study of the Child* (Vol. 3, 1949) pp. 333-352.

Chapter One

Autism: Finding a Definition

Understand

I want people to understand
I know it's hard to do
I think they can, if they try.
Understand, won't you?

Understanding is so hard
I long to see it real
I just hope, really hope
It's not a lost ideal.
David Eastham[4]

When people first become involved with autism, whether as parents, teachers, family members, caregivers or professionals, they are struck by the lack of readily available information on this subject. Accessible material is often filled with confusion as well as a variety of contradictions and discrepancies. The lack of agreement on this subject is so critical that the different disputes by specialists are included as part of the definition for infantile autism in The Penguin Dictionary of Psychology.[5]

This lack of a universal definition of autism is extremely frustrating. The more we delve into the situation, the worse our dilemma becomes. Caught behind the confusion is a group of people no one knows much about, and therefore no one is able to help.

Dr. Leo Kanner first defined autism in 1943. Dr. Kanner noticed similarities among many of his patients. He found that these children all shared certain problem areas: relating with people and objects, communication, eating, a need for sameness, a tendency to be anxious around other people, repetitive behaviours, horror reactions to sensory over stimulation such as loud noises, and the lack of ability to reach out to be picked up.[6]

Since then, Kanner's description has been accepted by scientists as the description of the basic symptoms of autism. Various studies on autism have revealed new evidence resulting in the addition or subtraction of features from Kanner's original definition. For example, one of the changes made on Kanner's work is apparent in the pamphlet "*Fact Sheet on Autism*" by the United States Department of Health and Human Services. Established levels of mental retardation for autistic people have been determined.[7] Sixty percent of autistic patients have IQ scores below fifty, twenty percent between fifty and seventy, and twenty percent greater than seventy. However, children do not test up to their abilities because these results are probably affected by the communication difficulties associated with autism. In spite of this, mental retardation has now become an accepted part of the puzzle to the point that the DSM-IV states that approximately 75% of children with Autistic Disorder function at a retarded level.[8]

To date, we have not determined the cause of autism. Various possible causes have been stressed throughout the world of psychology at different times, from the ridiculous theory of "cold refrigerator parents"[9] of the '50's and '60's to the current, most widely supported explanation, "brain dysfunction".[10] The specific area of the brain affected, or the reason for this dysfunction has a completely different focus depending on which specialist you talk to and where their particular realm of interest lies.

The diagnosis of autism is based on criteria set forth by the *Diagnostic and Statistical Manual of Mental Disorders, Fourth Edition*, better known as the DSM-IV.[11] This manual concentrates directly on the symptoms of autism, not on a cause or a cure.

According to the DSM-IV, the diagnostic criteria for autistic disorder includes:

A. A total of six (or more) items for (1), (2), and (3), with at least two from (1), and one each from (2) and (3).

(1) a qualitative impairment in social interaction as manifested by at least two of the following:

(a) marked impairment in the use of multiple nonverbal behaviors such as eye-to-eye gaze, facial expression, body posture, and gestures to regulate social interaction,

(b) failure to develop peer relationships appropriate to developmental level,

(c) a lack of spontaneous seeking to share enjoyment, interests or achievements with other people (e.g. by lack of showing, bringing, or pointing out objects of interest),

(d) lack of social or emotional reciprocity.

(2) qualitative impairments in communication as manifested by at least one of the following:

(a) delay in, or total lack of, the development of spoken language (not accompanied by an attempt to compensate through alternative modes of communication such as gesture or mime),

(b) in individuals with adequate speech, marked impairment in the ability to initiate or sustain a conversation with others,

(c) stereotyped and repetitive use of language or idiosyncratic language,

(d) lack of varied, spontaneous make-believe play or social imitative play appropriate to developmental level.

(3) restricted repetitive and stereotyped patterns of behavior, interests, and activities, as manifested by at least one of the following:

(a) encompassing preoccupation with one or more stereotyped and restricted patterns of interest that is abnormal either in intensity or focus,

(b) apparently inflexible adherence to specific, non-functional routines or rituals,

(c) stereotyped and repetitive motor mannerisms (e.g. hand or finger flapping or twisting, or complex whole body movements),

(d) persistent preoccupation with parts of objects.

B. Delays or abnormal functioning in at least one of the following areas, with onset prior to three years: (1) social interaction, (2) language as used in social communication, or (3) symbolic or imaginative play.

C. The disturbance is not better accounted for by Rett's Disorder or Childhood Disintegrative Disorder.[12]

As you will note, there is no mention of sensory over stimulation in the diagnostic criteria section of DSM-IV. However, there is brief comment under the title Associated Features and Disorders, where it is stated "there may be odd responses to sensory stimuli (e.g. a high threshold for pain, over sensitivity to sounds or being touched, exaggerated reactions to light or odors, fascination with certain stimuli)".[13] This is an improvement from the DSM-IIIR in which there was no mention at all of abnormal responses to sensations.[14]

For parents who have just learned they have an autistic child, the search for concrete and useful information on this subject is often even more frustrating and confusing than for the student or professional with access to psychological texts and scientific journals. Parents, who require access to accurate and useful information, find little through their medical practitioners or public libraries. If they are lucky, they are referred to local or national autism societies where collections of material on this subject are gradually growing. Again, material from these societies can be highly confusing and conflicting.

Examples of the changing definitions of autism can be seen within chapters of the Autism Society of America (ASA). In the 1993 pamphlet handed out by the Los Angeles Chapter of ASA[15], it states:

> AUTISM is a severely incapacitating lifelong developmental disability that typically appears during the first three years of life. It occurs in approximately fifteen out of every 10,000 births and is four times more common in boys than in girls. It has been found throughout the world in families of all racial, ethnic and social backgrounds. No known factors in the psychological environment of a child have been shown to cause autism.
>
> The symptoms, caused by disorders in the brain, include:
>
> · Disturbances in the development of physical, social and language skills.
>
> · Abnormal responses to sensations. Any one of or a combination of senses and responses may be affected: sight, hearing, touch, smell, taste, balance, reaction to pain and the way a child holds his head or body.
>
> · Absence or impairment of speech and language, although specific thinking capabilities may be present.
>
> · Abnormal ways of relating to people, objects and events.
>
> AUTISM occurs by itself or in association with other disorders such as viral infections, metabolic disturbances and epilepsy, which affects functioning of the brain.
>
> · It is important to distinguish autism from retardation or mental disorders, since diagnostic confusion may result in referral to inappropriate or ineffective treatment techniques.
>
> · The severe form of the syndrome may include self-injury, obsessive repetition, aggression and tantrums.
>
> AUTISM is treatable. Early diagnosis and intervention are vital to the future development of the child.

In contrast, let's look at a more current definition for autism as found in the pamphlet handed out by the South Central Pennsylvania Chapter of ASA in 1996.[16] It states:

> AUTISM is a developmental disability that typically appears during the first three years of life. The result of a neurological disorder that affects functioning of the brain, autism and its associated behaviors occur in approximately 15 out of every 10,000 individuals.
>
> Autism is four times more prevalent in boys than girls and knows no racial, ethnic or social boundaries. Family income, lifestyle or educational levels do not affect the chance of occurrence.

Autism interferes with the normal development of the brain in areas, which control verbal and nonverbal communication, social interaction, and sensory development. Children or adults with autism may exhibit repeated body movements such as hand flapping or rocking, show unusual responses to people or attachments to objects and resist changes in routine. In some cases aggressive behavior may be present. It is conservatively estimated that 400,000 people in the U.S. today have some form of autism. Its prevalence now makes it more common than Down's syndrome.

Since this ASA chapter also disseminates information on Pervasive Developmental Delay (PDD), another paragraph was added to their autism definition to explain the connection between the two terms.

Pervasive Developmental Delay (PDD) is a spectrum disorder, meaning the symptoms and characteristics can present themselves in a wide variety of combinations, from mild to severe. The more severe forms are referred to as Autism. Those who do not meet all the criteria for autism are diagnosed as PDD-NOS (not otherwise specified). However, autism serves as a useful model for all PDD, and it is reasonable to assume that most of the conceptual framework and scientific knowledge developed about autism will also apply to PDD or PDD-NOS.[17]

Parents who wish to search for further information may be referred to the Autism Services Center in Huntington, West Virginia or to The Autism Research Institute in San Diego, California. Parents of autistic children, who also specialize in this field as professionals, established both of these organizations.

Conflicting definitions are sent out by these last two organizations, demonstrating the unique position occupied by professionals in this field. Anyone is free to care for those with autism and carry out research using their own definitions as a basis of study.

Dr. Ruth Sullivan of the Autism Services Center claims her definition is based on personal and professional expertise in the field.[18] She states that the two essential features of autism are extreme aloneness and unresponsiveness to other people, probably based on the profound and pervasive inability to understand and use language in a normal way and preservation of sameness.[19]

Dr. Lorna Wing, of Great Britain, developed a second definition, sent out by the Autism Services Centre. She works from the premise that autism is a problem of understanding messages from the senses, especially sight and hearing. Although the eyes and ears of autistic children seem normal, it is believed that when visual and auditory messages reach the brain, they are not linked into an understandable picture of the outside world. This leads to a lack of understanding of speech and gesture and hence a lack of ability to communicate. Because of the missing link in understanding, autistic children appear to be withdrawn and seem to live in an isolated world of their own. Moreover, the frustration caused by the inability to communicate often leads to disturbed behaviour.[20]

Researchers in Great Britain have focused on this assumption where their present emphasis in autism is based on the "theory of mind".[21] This theory has led to a new definition from The National Autistic Society of Great Britain. In their pamphlet for professionals, they claim, "the primary problem underlying autism appears to affect a particular set of abilities that are innate in the rest of humanity. People who are autistic do not instinctively recognize themselves as being part of the human species; they lack intuitive understanding of people's thoughts, feelings and needs, and thus, are not able to respond to them appropriately."[22] The pamphlet then goes on to state that problems with socialization, communication, learning, and adapting as well as the repetitive stereotyped patterns of behaviour that they describe as secondary problems, can be traced back to this primary cause.

Dr. Rimland of the Autism Research Institute has also developed his own definition. He claims autism is:

> · A very severe behavioural disorder of childhood, which in most cases starts at birth, or soon after birth, and presents a major handicap to the individual for his or her entire life, although there have been a few unexpected cases of at least partial recovery. Autistic children are generally very well formed and physically attractive. Their disorder is difficult to characterize, but a very prominent feature is their inability to relate or communicate with other human beings in ways that are natural or meaningful. Some autistic children are mute and others do have speech, but it is usually of a rather bizarre, ritualistic type, which is not very well suited to communication.
>
> · An autistic child has been described as living in a dream world, in a glass ball, or in a world of his own. The cause is unknown, although it is known that the old-fashioned idea that autism is an emotional disorder is entirely incorrect. It is well known that autism is brought on by some metabolic dysfunction of the brain, but beyond that, the cause is not known.[23]

The ramifications of the combination of the lack of a unified framework of knowledge on autism as well as the apparent freedom to develop one's own definition of autism can be very disturbing. Anyone who chooses to come up with a theory is often free to care for those who have autism without set guidelines or effective monitoring systems. For example, a situation developed in Canada in which a psychologist developed a new theory on autism, based directly on her personal experiences of retraining her daughter, who had suffered brain damage in an automobile accident. Based on her background and current belief of "brain dysfunction", the psychologist determined that people with autism are out of control and need to learn control. She went on to develop and institute a program of care focused directly on teaching clients how to control themselves. Until the clients learned this control, the staff was responsible to provide control through the use of physical restraint.

In extreme situations, this program depended on physical strength and confrontations between clients and staff. It can be a very short step from physical control to physical abuse. Allegations of abuse quickly surfaced and investigations were carried out. A limited amount of working knowledge of autism was available in the province, so no one was willing to challenge the unique theory and method of treatment developed by this psychologist. As there were no other options available, many desperate parents supported the program. For a dozen years, clients endured what could only be termed torture. Thankfully, enough evidence of the physical abuse was brought to light to have the whole operation shut down, but not before one lad had the misfortune of losing his life.

Regrettably, this is only one example of questionable treatment for people who suffer with autism. The use of electric cattle prods, practices associated with some behaviour modification programs seeking to eliminate undesirable behaviours, and the administration of a variety of psychotic drugs have been based on other theories with little regard for the actual feelings of the clients, or any long term effects they might suffer. The need for caution is very apparent.

Do the Senses Play a Part?

The examples of different definitions of autism offer little insight to the puzzling contradictions of sensory response, as noted in the introduction of this book. To date, scientists and professionals may make brief reference to the senses or ignore them altogether. No one seems to be very interested in questioning the role they may play in this syndrome.

How fascinating it is to look at another source and find an opposite reaction. According to individuals with autism, their disability is linked directly to the senses. They describe how the touch of another human being can be excruciating, how smells can be overpowering, how hearing certain sounds can hurt, how sight is distorted, and how tastes are too strong.[24] The world of the person with autism is often a world of pain. The development of the autistic personality is their method of coping with this pain.

Individual descriptions may be questioned as to their scientific validity and objectivity, but in a field that is already so confusing and frustrating, I believe the similarities of these descriptions are definitely worth noting.

The Individuals with Autism Say .....

> · Now the reason that children withdraw is because of sensory problems. Loud noises just hurt my ears. When a loud noise goes off, I put my hands over my ears. It hurts. People touched me. It was like a tidal wave of stimulation. On an autistic child a scratchy petticoat will feel like sandpaper just scratching her raw. Her skin is oversensitive, and my hearing - certain sounds will just blast through my ears. You're so overwhelmed by the defect in the sensory system that all you want to do is withdraw because it just hurts. How can I be thinking of emotions when I'm just trying to protect myself from this terrible noise onslaught?[25]

> · For me, my expressive difficulties were secondary and sprang from these primary inconsistencies in my perception of the world around me and in the complex psychological defence systems I created to compensate, which trapped me even more. Sensorially, this can mean that any one of a combination of the senses can become extremely acute. For me, this made some high-pitched sounds intolerable, and bright light became either intolerable or mesmerizing. Touch was, as always, intolerable.[26]

> · i didnt enjoy the drive today at all i cant stand any more and then i switch off i cant stand the impressions its obvious i cant avoid trouble every sound hurts me i can bear a sound like singing or whispering inside a room but i cant get rid of exhausting talking it makes me crazy it is nonsense to believe in a cure i cant bear chattering in the street any more than i ever could i felt silly today when a well dressed lady asked how to get to eisenacher street i was anxious because she asked for information they all turn around and look at me for reasons i dont understand i am always afraid of people and i act stupid because then people will leave me in peace.[27] (Note: B. Sellin chooses to type without capitals and punctuation marks.)

> · I see autism as a neurochemical disorder that is both difficult to diagnose and impossible to easily understand. There are, however, as I see it, some definite commonalties among people regarded as autistic. The commonalties I've observed are as follows:
>
> 1. Extreme sensitivity in the areas of sight, sound, touch, taste and smell.

2. Overly developed brain reactions to stimuli in these areas.
3. Motor planning difficulties and anomalies.
4. Need for structure and resistance to change to avoid confusing and already overloaded neural receptors.
5. Excessive motor activity and/or anxiety reactions and/or withdrawal-avoidance behaviours to compensate for and/or adapt to excessive input of information.
6. Great powers of observation and keen powers of recall for visual and/or auditory stimuli.

> I would like to say at this point that I disagree with much of what professionals think they know about autism and people with autism. Most of us are not retarded, we both have and comprehend feelings, we are capable of both imagination and abstract thinking, and we experience pain, pleasure, sadness, and joy. While it may seem that we don't understand things, this is not true. The real difficulties occur in speed and style of processing, digesting, and responding to what has been presented.[28]

The word autism comes from the roots `aut' and `ism'. These root words indicate a tendency to be involved with oneself or a condition in which one is totally absorbed in one's apprehensions of the world. Autism implies, therefore, a pathological state in which the internal state of the person is not connected to reality.[29]

If we take the vivid descriptions reported by those with autism into account, we have to admit that our reality does not match their reality. If our reality does not indicate a pathological inner problem, perhaps theirs does not either. Their feelings and experiences are as real and meaningful to them as ours are to us. Perhaps it is time to listen to those who have autism and come up with a new definition based on their descriptions.

In the early seventies, Carl Delacato promoted a revolutionary approach to autism.[30] He determined that the abnormal behaviour of children with autism was tied to their sensory response and used two terms, "hypo" and "hyper" to measure the different levels of stimulation. Sensory systems were labelled hypo sensitive if there was little or no response to stimulation and were labelled hypersensitive when an extreme response occurred after stimulation. Delacato claims that his work with those who measured hyper went very well, but there was not the same progress made with those who were considered hypo.[31] As his ideas spread, it became acceptable to characterize the sensory responses of individuals with autism as "mixed up".[32]

There are two problems with this assumption. In the first place, "mixed up" does not match what those who have autism are actually saying. Furthermore, how can anyone ever develop a therapy that begins with a statement of "mixed up"? As the reports by individuals with autism indicate, as well as the success rate that Delacato had with those he measured at the hyper level, one may assume we have to concentrate on the area of super sensitivity. Perhaps the clients who measured hypo were indeed on the hyper scale, but far beyond the level Delacato was measuring. Because of their extreme reaction to sensory stimulation, it became vital to deaden their sensory response system continuously, and thus they appeared to have what was termed the hypo response.

Biochemical Clues

In order to understand how and why autistic individuals respond as they do, we must look at what happens to each of us when our senses are stimulated. Stimulation from our environment enters the brain in various forms, such as sound waves through our ears, or light waves through the retina of our eyes. Our nervous system passes this information through the brain and body by the use of biochemical neurotransmitters. The amount of stimulation, which is passed through the system, is determined by the amount of neurotransmitter processed in each neuron.

Dopamine beta hydroxylase is the biochemical, which is released from sympatic nerve endings during stimulation.[33] An increase in neural activity or stimulation results in an increase in the level of this enzyme.[34] When the autistic individual experiences an overwhelming response to environmental stimulation, high levels of dopamine beta hydroxylase will move through the system.[35] Studies have measured dopamine levels in different subject groups, and research indicates that autistic children have higher levels of plasma dopamine beta hydroxylase than normal subjects.[36] The highest levels in one study were found in the subgroup labelled "retarded autistic subjects".[37]

Homovanillic acid is the final product in the metabolism of dopamine beta hydroxylase. Higher levels of urinary homovanillic acid reflects increased dopamine metabolism in the central nervous system.[38] Studies have found that autistic subjects have higher levels of urinary homovanillic acid and that these levels are even higher when the subjects are both autistic and mentally retarded.[39]

Homovanillic acid levels have also been found to be higher in the cerebrospinal fluid of autistic subjects when compared to normal levels.[40] In comparison studies between autistic twins, the twin who is considered more disturbed and has more severe behaviour problems has been found to have the higher level of homovanillic acid in his cerebrospinal fluid.[41]

Neuroleptics, drugs that block dopamine receptors in the brain, have been administered to autistic subjects. This can result in the elimination of much of the abnormal patterns of autistic behaviour such as repetition, aggression and self-mutilation.[42] On the other hand, stimulants produce the opposite reaction. Stimulants are so named because they increase the level of dopamine released during neural activity. Administration of stimulant medication to autistic children causes extreme agitation, hypersensitivity to sensory input, and head banging to the point that these children are described as "climbing the walls".[43]

From the high levels of dopamine beta hydroxylase measured in the systems of autistic individuals, we may assume that the level of stimulation experienced by those who have autism is higher than that of normal people. These results also validate the vivid descriptions of extreme feelings, which have been shared by the autistic population.

Habituation is the natural response of the human body to sensory stimulation in which the brain gradually ignores a stimulus until there is no response to that stimulation.[44] An example of this reaction is our response as we enter an apartment and notice a certain odour. After a period of time in the apartment, we do not even realize the odour still exists, unless we leave and return later. Habituation does not normally occur if the stimulation is traumatic or has a reward involved.

Individuals with autism take a much longer time to habituate to a stimulus than normal people.[45] This is likely due to their high level of response to stimulation. To a normal person, the stimulation may not be threatening. To the autistic individual with high acuity, the same amount of stimulation may well cause pain or discomfort.

Sensitization is the opposite response to habituation and happens when a threat is perceived from a stimulus.[46] Sensitization occurs when a person reacts strongly to a response that leads one to react more strongly to similar stimuli in the near future.

Sensitization causes greater amounts of calcium ions to be released into the neural terminals during stimulation. The increase in calcium ions results directly in the release of more neurotransmitters throughout the system. This in turn increases the level of feeling or response. Effects of sensitization and habituation can last for minutes, or up to weeks, in a normal population, depending on the original stimulus.

High acuity to sensory stimulation may well lead autistic people to a constant state of sensitization. The already high levels of sensitivity may appear sharper. They may also appear to increase over time. Negative behaviours may occur with less and less stimulation.

Another biochemical that modulates neural activity in the brain is serotonin.[47] Serotonin is manufactured in the pineal gland of the brain[48] and production is directly affected by visual stimulation. Studies indicate that increased levels of light, such as those found in summer as compared to winter, lead to increased levels of production.[49] Serotonin is found in higher levels in autistic subjects when compared to normal subjects.[50] This may well indicate a higher level of response to visual stimulation (light waves entering the retina) from the environment.[51]

Endorphins belong to a family of chemicals that was first discovered at the University of Aberdeen[52] in 1975. At first, production was measured in caged animals engaged in stereotyped behaviours such as pacing or chewing the bars -- much like the repetitive behaviours of the autistic individuals. An increased level of repetitious behaviours leads to an increase in the amount of endorphins in the brain.

Later research concentrated on the role of endorphins both in animals and man. In human beings, studies indicate that the presence of these peptides influence neurons throughout the central nervous system by depressing the response. In other words, when endorphins are present, the amount of sensory reaction is decreased in the brain.[53] However, in one section of the brain, the hippocampus, this response is the opposite. In the hippocampus, the presence of endorphins leads to such a high level of response that seizures are induced. Although this response may seem contradictory, it is not. The neurons involved in the hippocampus are inhibitory; therefore depressing their ability to react produces excitement.

The level of endorphins found in individuals with autism is higher than that for normal subjects.[54] Autistic individuals may also suffer epileptic seizures, which could originate in the hippocampus of the brain.[55]

Other indications of a state of hyper arousal in autistic subjects have been documented. These include electroencephalographic evidence of low-voltage EEG irregular behaviour,[56] increased peripheral blood flow during performance tests,[57] and generally elevated cerebral metabolism indicated by the Positron Emission Tomography results.[58]

These biochemical clues lead directly to one conclusion. Individuals with autism definitely experience sensation at a higher level than other people. This evidence supports the vivid descriptions of those who have autism.

Normal Response to Over Stimulation

In 1975, Z. Lipowski reviewed studies based on over stimulation of the sensory systems of normal people.[59] The review included research, which focused on a single sensory experience such as noise, as well as those using a combination of stimulation such as light, electric shock, and loud music. Reported effects included withdrawal, disorganized thinking, aggression, anxiety, fatigue, distorted body images, and what was described as autistic thoughts and behaviour.[60] Extremely high levels of stimulation, from which one could not escape, led rapidly to sleep.[61] The actual number of studies carried out in this area is limited and will likely not increase substantially due to the ethical problems of subjecting people to over stimulation.

Again the descriptions of autistic individuals match these scientific results. When "normal" human beings are over stimulated, they resort to autistic-like behaviour. Thus we could assume that the symptoms of autism are directly caused by over stimulation from the environment.

Hyperacusis

> Imagine living in a world where the volume is always turned all the way up. Where the snap, crackle, pop of your breakfast cereal sounds like firecrackers exploding. Where autumn leaves crunching under your feet sound like shattering glass. Where the water running from a faucet is louder than Niagara Falls.[62]

So begins an article on hyperacusis, a rare condition where people who experience normal hearing for most of their lives, suddenly become hypersensitive to sound. This usually occurs as a result of exposure to extremely loud sudden noises, repeated exposure to loud noises, or in some instances as the result of using certain medications. This intolerance to sound makes it difficult to hold a job, socialize, or gain much enjoyment from life. For some with hyperacusis, earplugs, earmuffs, and noise suppressors have allowed the sufferers to take part in ordinary activities. However, others have been driven to give up everything they love and build special insulated quarters in their homes to escape the noise.

It is interesting to note that many of the descriptions of the experience of hyperacusis mirror those of people with autism. However, their history of normal hearing gives them something to compare their current lives to, as well as giving them the ability to communicate far more clearly with us. For example:

> It's hard for me to say just when certain noises started to bother me. I can only remember that about 15 years ago my good hearing started to become even more acute. I could hear sounds of people approaching the house, the sounds of traffic blocks away, planes and trains miles off and numerous other sounds long before others in the same room could. Gradually, these became more pronounced and closer sounds around me became more annoying. About 5 years ago, more sounds became distressingly harder to bear and I found myself trying to escape by distancing myself from the worst offenders.
>
> I gave up playing the organ, quit my bell-ringing choir and stopped attending the symphony... since music was one of my greatest joys; this has made me truly sad. I can still enjoy radio, TV or CDs if the volume is low. Traveling presents some problems as well. When we travel, I'm sure I drive hotel managers crazy by insisting on the most isolated room - away from the ice machine, the elevator, noisy heaters or air conditioners. We travel less and I become more selective as I try to adapt.

My worst problems at home are the refrigerator, electric fan noises, outside traffic, vibrating sounds, delivery trucks and cars with blaring radios. My computer motor and fan I can tolerate, probably because the tower is on the carpeted floor and I play background music to mask the sound. We live three blocks from a Military Academy. Their morning reveille, frequent drills, march cadences and parade music, plus weekend outdoors sports cheers, band music and canons going off every touchdown are a real daytime problem.[63]

Now not only do loud sounds bother me but regular sounds bother me. I mean when I talk it echoes and hurts my ears. There is a feeling of fullness in my head and sometimes my ears hurt even when I am not around sound. There is always this feeling of pain, which starts in my ears and creates headaches. I am real fidgety and nervous with high anxiety. Every time I listen to somebody or talk it just drains me. The worse thing is my friends, the doctors, as well as my family think I am crazy. I have never felt so alone in my life and no one understands.[64]

Noises that were mildly offensive before are violating now. I put in my earplugs as soon as I get off the train in the morning in Manhattan and do not remove them until I am inside a building. I do not attend weddings, concerts, loud parties, and many of the fun things young people my age do without a thought. I am careful of what movies I see, and always have earplugs on hand in case I get caught in a loud situation. I walk everyday to exercise and de-stress....I've attempted weddings and sporting events to try and live a normal life, but the sound makes my head vibrate and the pain is unbearable. Barking dogs, clanking dishes and even the sounds of some cars are painful.[65]

When we consider the descriptions by people with hyperacusis, we have the opportunity to become aware of what those people with autism who experience extreme sensitivity to sound, may be experiencing in their day-to-day lives. This is not something that can be brushed easily aside. It is an overriding condition, which controls every thought, and choice a person makes each day. Withdrawal from society, the common reaction of people with autism, is also that of people who suffer from hyperacusis. Hyperacusis gives us another window to observe the effects of over stimulation on "normal" people. Their experience gives us an opportunity to make sense of the reactions of those with autism to the noisy world in which we live.

A Sensory Theory of Autism

The senses of the individual are very acute. The human body is not designed to deal effectively with such acuity; thus, stimulation results in pain. The human body has biochemical means to deal with pain (endorphins), which result in the blockage of not only the pain, but also the senses.

The behaviour of the autistic individual is tied directly to the reaction of his or her acute sensitivity. Individuals with autism may protect themselves from the pain of over stimulation by withdrawal. Examples of withdrawal include resisting hugs or physical contact, closing one's eyes, walking on tiptoes, and so on. Through the release of endorphins, the person with autism is able to create protection from the pain. Endorphins can be created by the repetition of behaviours such as rocking, pacing, twirling objects, and flapping hands. Those who have autism may also purposely overload their sensory system in order to shut it down. For example, they may stare directly into a bright light, scream loudly, or mutilate themselves by biting or head banging.

The sensory system matures over time. The greatest problems with the acuity of senses occur in infancy and childhood. When mature, sensory response to stimulation may have diminished to a point that it is no longer as painful, but the need for protection, which the individual has lived with since birth, has not allowed the individual to develop like the rest of our population. The person continues to live in a state of anxiety, waiting for the pain to return. Any feeling is regarded as a threat and the body protects itself by overreacting or by becoming dead. Those who have autism need to be taught that it is safe to have feelings. Years of exposure to over stimulation have resulted in damage to the sensory system; for example, damaged nerves in the ears that affect the individual's response.

Autism may be the normal human reaction to acute sensitivity and over stimulation. Those who have autism are not *dis*abled, they are *super*abled. The natural, human means of dealing with this super ability results in a developmental disability. Differences in the autistic population can be attributed to the level of sensory difficulty, the number of senses involved, and the different environments to which individuals are exposed. Statistically, the amount of variation is unlimited. Differences can also be attributed to individual variances as found throughout the normal population.

Although the current view of most scientists is that autism is caused by brain dysfunction, I believe it is not a dysfunction, but instead a difference in brain physiology which is directly affected by genetics. Different response levels to stimulation have been measured in subjects who were labelled introverts and extroverts by Hans Eysenck.[66] This work has also been carried out by Jerome Kagan, using the terms inhibited and uninhibited.[67] Both researchers have discovered there is a definite difference in the physiological makeup of human beings who measure introverted or extroverted. In the experiments on over stimulation, extroverts were found to have higher tolerance levels to stimulation than introverts.[68] In time, I feel that we will find that autism is the extreme response on the inhibited or introverted scales.[69]

The Population Sample

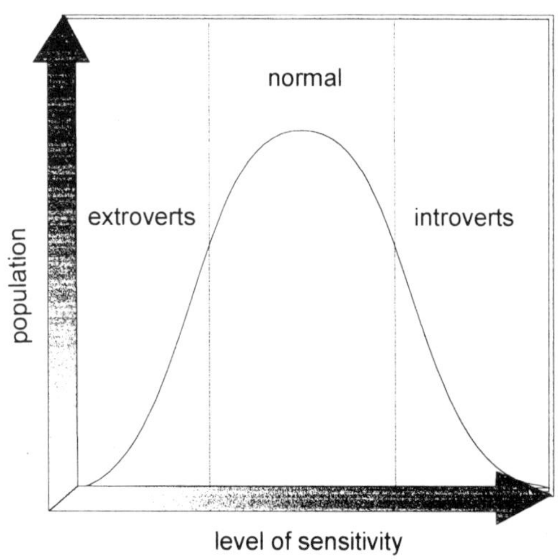

People with autism would be found on the extreme high end of the sensitivity scale, with those diagnosed with PDD-NOS and Asperger's at a slightly lower level of sensitivity, placing them on the continuum of human life. Autism becomes a "difference" rather than a "disorder".

Thus, we are not talking about brain dysfunction, but a difference in brain physiology that makes up a natural population sample. The low percentage of people with autism indicates they will be found on the extreme end of the sensitivity bell curve.

Program of Care

In developing a program of care for people with autism, the recognition of a painful existence caused by stimuli in the environment is of prime consideration. Super sensitivity to sound, smell, touch, sight, taste, and emotion means that the environment we share with people with autism, without ourselves experiencing sensory discomfort, may cause them extreme pain. Caregivers must be aware of this reality and be prepared to deal with their own behaviour and attitudes, as much as they deal with the environment, behaviours and attitudes of those who have autism. Even if one cannot empathize with the individual with autism the fact that we are trying our best to understand makes an incredible difference. Signs to watch for and methods of care for each of the five senses as well as stereotyped behaviours, obsessions, social interaction, communication, and intelligence are outlined throughout the following chapters. I close this chapter with some generalizations that are applicable to all the senses.

The most important aspect of this program is to share all information directly with the individual with autism. Those who have autism are very aware that they are different, but they have never known *how* they are different.[70] They assume that everyone else feels just like they do but has better methods of coping, in much the same way that we attribute their feelings and expereince to be the same as ours.[71] By sharing the experiences of others with autism and describing how these descriptions are different from our own experiences, we can reach even those who seem totally beyond our scope. The most amazing thing about this program is how little time it takes to get through to individuals with autism.

It is very important to tell children who have autism what is wrong with them. Thomas McKean was an adult before he searched through past medical records to find out why he was different.[72] Sean Barron discovered autism in a classroom in high school. At the time he wondered why the teacher was so cruel as to describe him in this way to his classmates.[73] Later he watched the movie *Son Rise* with his mother and finally was told that he was autistic.[74] Due to some of the "hopeless" descriptions of autism, many parents and professionals believe they are protecting the children by not sharing this information with them. Instead, they are withholding the truth and thus creating a situation in which the children imagine that they are worthless or bad.[75] Imagination can make things far more difficult than does real life.

Garth has had trouble sleeping from the time he was first brought home. His parents were tired and irritated after coping with years of disturbed sleep, but were unable to find a remedy. When I first came in contact with them, I suggested that they share the words of other autistic individuals with their child, and also correlate his actual behaviour with sensitivity to sensation. Instances of acute hearing and an ability to see in the dark had been described to me. The parents spent an evening sharing this information with their four-year-old son. Garth slept through the whole night for the first time in his life. Later the parents phoned me to report that they had just gone through three weeks of undisturbed sleep. By allowing this child to perceive his actual differences and sharing with him the knowledge that he was not alone in feeling this way, we also allowed him the freedom to relax and find himself acceptable.

Mark is a 29-year-old male, presently living in a group home. Seventeen years of his life were spent in an institution where he was often the victim of severe physical abuse. He feels safe in this home but he is very leery of strangers.

I came into the home to explain this program to the staff, insisting, as I always do, that the autistic client be present to hear what I had to say. Mark was very agitated when I arrived, pacing up and down the floor, twiddling his fingers, pausing now and then to pull his pants down, and then up. He stayed in the adjoining room and paced as I began my talk. As time passed he gradually began to relax. First the pants routine disappeared, then the finger twiddling, and finally the pacing. After about an hour he came and sat on the chair next to me and watched me intently. He reached out, took my hand, and began to stroke his chin with it. As he has bitten staff members in the past, I resisted his movements. He then took my hand and gently rested it against my chin. I had no idea what was going on and tried to continue my presentation. The young man became very agitated and actually ripped the drapes off the window behind us.

The staff members had no explanation for this extreme behaviour. Soon, an afternoon worker arrived and related an incident that had happened a couple of days before. Mark had fallen at the swimming pool and cut his inner lip. The worker had forgotten to tell anyone, or to note the injury in the daily log. We checked Mark's mouth and found he had a severe infection. Needless to say, the rest of my presentation was forgotten as we rushed him to an emergency clinic.

As one reviews this situation, one might note that what could have been described as bizarre behaviour for no discernible reason was discovered instead to be an attempt by this young man to communicate a problem. He rarely made any effort to communicate with anyone and usually hid when strangers were present. However, on this day, it only took the description of this program to give Mark the confidence not only to try to communicate, but to do so with a total stranger.

Sharing the common experiences of people with autism with those who are high- functioning can also have a dramatic impact on their lives. Darren White is one of the first young men I contacted who had chosen to share his past. Although he had succeeded in coping with daily life in our society and becoming self-sufficient, he still had a terrible time-sharing his feelings and experiences with anyone, even his parents. Since we do not recognize and accept the actual feelings of those who have autism from birth, it becomes extremely difficult for them to ever share what they truly feel.

In 1986, with a lot of effort and patience, Darren was able to describe some of his childhood experiences to his parents.[76] After I had read his biography, I wrote a letter to his mother describing this program and the theories I was developing. In the letter, I stated that I do not believe that autism is a disability, but instead see it as a super ability.

When I met Darren in person, he told me "this one line had changed my life completely. No longer do I have to hide away from the world, feeling inferior." While in England, I had the opportunity to speak at a school and was pleased to have Darren present. As I watched him, sitting calmly, discussing his feelings and experiences with the teachers, I couldn't help thinking how far he had come in two years.

A teacher reports that she took this advice to heart after reading *Autism: Handle with Care*. She worked in a classroom with eleven children with autism. As one can well imagine, with this many students in the room, it was rarely calm and peaceful. However, the chaos ceased while she shared the words of those with autism with her students. She chose only to read the portions from *Autism: Handle with Care*, which are direct quotes from people with autism. As she read, all of the students sat quietly at their desks, listening intently to the words. Some relaxed to the point that they folded their arms on their desks and rested their heads on them. It was an experience she will always remember. Never before had the students responded so well to anything she had shared with them.

When one recognizes that stimulation causes problems for people with autism, it may be tempting to eliminate all stimulation in order to protect the individual. This choice is by no means appropriate. Due to the ability, and the necessity, to block out the world, those who have autism have missed out on much of the stimulation of normal development. In order to catch up with the rest of the population, they may need more stimulation than most. However, this stimulation must be carried out in an environment that is safe; where lights are dim, voices low, and touch is soft and fleeting. By providing a safe environment, the child is given the opportunity to learn and to respond appropriately.

In times of extreme stress, a totally stimuli-free environment may be useful so that the individual has the opportunity to calm down. At a school in Alberta, Canada, a time-out room in a neutral colour and with soft, padded walls was installed. Teachers used it for the first couple of years after the school opened. As they watched students with autism, who were wild and uncontrolled in the classroom, sit quietly in the middle of this room and do nothing, they assumed the room was a waste of space. Unfortunately it was removed from the school and the children with autism no longer have anywhere to go to calm down, for that is what they were doing as they sat quietly. When the students did not exhibit behaviours that fit the pattern expected by the teachers (throwing themselves up against the padded walls to vent their frustrations), the false assumption was made that nothing productive was happening.

Individuals with autism must also have access to the normal environment we all inhabit, in order to develop socially and learn to cope with the real world. This access gives them the chance to become full members of society. As caregivers, we must realize that the ability to learn factual information in this environment may be limited. Learning to cope with the flow of stimulation will take precedence over acquiring skills or knowledge. By recognizing the need to supply both stimulus-free and normal environments, we can help those with autism to grow and develop to the best of their abilities.

When working with an autistic person, we must realize that we are not only dealing with the present situation, but also with a history, which is very present in the person's memory. In the past, it was believed that because of an inability to play imaginative games, individuals with autism had little or no memory. This assumption is totally inaccurate. In fact, due to their need to protect themselves and their attempts to constantly control their environments, those who have autism have better memories than most of us. When we are working with a client and the agitation exhibited makes absolutely no sense at all to us, perhaps we are dealing with the memory of a past experience. The agitation is very real and must be recognized as such. Since sharing their feelings is such a problem, there are times that we, as caretakers, may only have empathy and a willingness to admit our lack of understanding to use as beneficial techniques. The lack of information can be a big part of the frustration of working with these clients. As long as we respect their feelings, even if we may not understand them, our work will be easier.

We were traveling with a nine-year old from one group home to another. Throughout the trip, he seemed relaxed, happy and showed few signs of agitation. We arrived at the other group home, the headquarters of this organization. As we walked into the main building, Daniel began flapping his hands at a furious rate, went up on his tiptoes and paced around the room quickly. We were completely puzzled by this abrupt change in behaviour.

It took a month before I pieced the story together. As I was talking to one of the workers from headquarters, she commented on how much this child had improved since he first joined the program. At that time they were building the kitchen cabinets in the main house. This child screamed for three weeks straight as they held him forcefully in the same room where electric saws were being used. The workers had absolutely no idea of his super sensitivity to sound. The torture, which they inadvertently forced him to endure, was not forgotten by this child and showed up as extreme agitation every time we took him into this building.

In this program of care, the biggest problem is changing the attitudes of the caregivers. The need to produce "normal people" who are "just like me" proves to be an insurmountable wall to many. Accepting that those who have autism are indeed different and that it is quite all right to experience things differently from you or me is a big step that many of us are not willing to take. [Those of you who have been frustrated trying to change autistic behaviour and think that those who have autism are stubborn, should take up the challenge of changing the behaviour of a professional or a therapist. It's a human difficulty.]

A word of caution is also in order. Once these ideas are shared with individuals with autism, seeds of hope are planted. Hope that can be dashed by stubborn and unthinking caregivers. Loss of apparent understanding may well lead to increased frustration on the part of the individual with autism, which will likely be exhibited in the form of more extreme behaviours.

I spoke to a group of teachers who eagerly accepted the ideas presented in this book and took them back to their classroom just before Christmas. Their students with autism began to respond immediately. After the Christmas break I talked to one of these teachers. She reported that they were having problems they had never experienced before with one girl. This student appeared to be extremely frustrated and angry at all times. I asked the teacher what change had occurred. She could not determine any cause and said "We're not doing anything different than we have done for the last three years." Over the Christmas holidays the teachers had all forgotten the effects of over stimulation on their students and had comfortably slipped back into their usual patterns of teaching. The student had not forgotten.

Choosing to ignore this information means choosing to ignore the individual with autism. No matter how much we want to help, no matter what background we have in the care of the disabled, no matter how much we demand, or how many hours we are willing to dedicate to the cause, if we ignore the super sensitivity to stimulation, we are ignoring the real person with whom we are dealing. It is our choice as providers of care to either make a real difference, or not.

4 David Eastham, *Understand* (Ottawa, Ontario: Oliver Pate, 1985) p. 5.

5 Arthur Reber, *The Penguin Dictionary of Psychology* (London: Penguin Books, 1985) p. 71.

6 Leo Kanner, "Autistic disturbances of affective contact," in *Classic Readings in Autism*, Anne Donnellan, ed. (New York: Teacher's College Press, 1985) pp. 41-48.

7 *Fact Sheet on Autism* (U.S. Department on Health and Human Services Publication #81-1877, 1980).

8 American Psychiatric Association, Diagnostic and Statistical Manual of Mental Disorders, Fourth Edition (Washington, D.C., 1994) p.67.

9 Bruno Bettelheim, *The Empty Fortress: Infantile Autism and the Birth of Self* (New York: The Free Press, 1972).

10 Paul Gabriel, "Educational techniques offer hope for autistic children", *The Grande Prairie Daily Herald Tribune* (September 16, 1992) p. 9.

11 The American Psychiatric Association, pp. 65-71.

12 The American Psychiatric Association, pp. 70-71

13 The American Psychiatric Association, pp. 67-68.

14 Edward Ornitz, "Autism: a disorder of directed attention", *Brain Dysfunction*, (Vol.1, 1988) p.309.

15 *Autism* (Los Angeles, California: The Los Angeles Chapter of the Autism Society of America, 3975 Landmark Street, Culver City, California, 90232).

16 *Autism and Pervasive Developmental Delay (PDD)* (New Freedom, Pennsylvania: South Central PA Chapter of the Autism Society of America, RD #32, Box 354, Mt. Airy Rd., New Freedom, Pennsylvania 17349).

17 Ibid.

18 Ruth Sullivan, *Definition of Autism* (Huntington, West Virginia: Autism Services Center, 1988) p. 1.

19 Ruth Sullivan, p. 2.

20 Lorna Wing, *Autism* (London: British National Society for Autistic Children, 1973). Provided by the Autism Services Center, Huntington, West Virginia.

21 Christopher Gilberg, "Treatment of Epilepsy in Autism" *Journal of Autism and Developmental Disorders* (Vol. 21, no. 1, 1991) pp. 61-77.

22 *What is Autism?* (London: The National Autistic Society, Great Britain). Professional advice from Lorna Wing and Michael Connelly.

23 Bernard Rimland ,"On Autism: an interview" (San Diego, California: Autism Research Institute).

24 Supporting evidence for these statements will be found throughout the book. See the section on each sense for matching quotes.

25 Temple Grandin on Debra Dimaio & Jim McPharlin, "Autistic Savants", *The Oprah Winfrey Show*, transcript (Chicago: Harpo Productions, January 10, 1989) p. 11.

26 Donna Williams, *Nobody Nowhere* (Toronto: Doubleday Canada Limited, 1992) p. 207.

27 Birger Sellin, *I don't want to be inside me anymore* (New York: Basic Books, 1995) pp. 142-143.

28 Sharisa Kochmeister, "Autism and Auditory Integration Training - My Viewpoint" in *Dancing in the Rain*, edited by Annabel Stehli (Westport, Connecticut: The Georgiana Organization, Inc., 1995) pp. 85-86.

29 Arthur Reber, *The Penguin Dictionary of Psychology* (London: Penguin Books, 1985) p. 70.

30 Carl Delacato, *The Ultimate Stranger The Autistic Child* (Novato, California: Academic Therapy Publications, 1974).

31 Carl Delacato, (an update).

32 Annabel Stehli, *The Sound of a Miracle* (New York: Doubleday, 1991) p. 188.

33 Irwin Kopin, Seymour Kaufman, Humberto Viveros, David Jacobwitz, Raymond Lake, Michael Zeigler, Walter Lovenberg, and Fred Goodwin, "Dopamine-beta-hydroxylase basic and clinical studies", *Annals of Internal Medicine* (Vol. 85, no. 2, 1976) p. 214.

34 Irwin Kopin, Seymour Kaufman, Humberto Viveros, David Jacobwitz, Raymond Lake, Michael Zeigler, Walter Lovenberg, and Fred Goodwin, p. 217.

35 C. Garnier, E. Comoy, C. Barthlemay, I. Leddet, B. Garreau, J. Muh and G. Lelord, "Dopamine-beta-hydroxylase (DBH) and Homovanillic Acid (HVA) in autistic children" *Journal of Autism and Developmental Disorders* (Vol. 16, no. 1, 1986) p. 28.

36 Robert Belmaker, Jocelyn Hattab and Richard Ebstein, "Plasma dopamine-beta-hydroxylase in childhood psychosis" *Journal of Autism and Childhood Schizophrenia* (Vol.8, no.3, 1978) p. 295.

37 C. Garnier, E. Comoy, C. Barthlemay, I. Leddet, B. Garreau, J. Muh and G. Lelord, p. 27.

38 B. Garreau, C. Barthlemay, J. Jouve, N. Bruneau, J. Muh and G. Lelord, "Urinary homovanillic acid levels of autistic children" *Developmental Medicine and Child Neurology* (Vol. 30), 1988) p. 93.

39 B. Garreau, C. Barthlemay, J. Jouve, N. Bruneau, J. Muh and G. Lelord, p. 96.

40 J. Gerald Young, Mary Ellen Kavanaugh, George Anderson, Bennett Shaywitz and Donald Cohen, "Clinical Neurochemistry of autism and associated disorders" *Journal of Autism and Developmental Disorders* (Vol. 12, no. 2, 1982) p. 153.

41 D. Cohen, B. Caparulo, B. Shaywitz and M. Bowers, "Dopamine and serotonin metabolism in neuropsychiatrically disturbed children: CFS homovanillic acid and 5-hydroxyindoleacetic acid" *Archives of General Psychiatry* (Vol. 34, no. 5, 1977) pp. 546-547.

42 J. Gerald Young, Mary Ellen Kavanaugh, George Anderson, Bennett Shaywitz and Donald Cohen, p. 153.

43 D. Janowsky, M. El-Yosef, J. Davis, and H. Sekerke, "Provocation of schizophrenic symptoms by intravenous administration of methylphenidate," *Archives of General Psychiatry* (Vol. 28., no. 2, 1978) pp. 185-191.

44 Stephen Kosslyn and Olivier Koenig, *Wet Mind* (New York: The Free Press, 1992) p. 384.

45 Karl Reichelt, personal correspondence. Based on Karl Reichelt, G. Saelid, T Lindback and J.B. Boler, "Childhood autism: a complex disorder," *Biological Psychiatry* (Vol. 21, 1986) pp. 1279-1290.

46 Stephen Kosslyn and Olivier Koenig, pp. 384-385.

47 J. Gerald Young, Mary Ellen Kavanaugh, George Anderson, Bennett Shaywitz and Donald Cohen, p. 148.

48 Bruce Fellman, "A clockwork gland," *Science* 85 (Vol.6, no. 4, 1985) p. 79.

49 M. Sheerd and G. Aghajanian, "Stimulation of medbrain raphe neuron: behavioral effcts of serotonin release" *Life Sciences* (Vol. 7, 1968) pp. 19-29.

50 E. Ritvo and B.J. Freeman, "A medical model of autism; etiology, pathology and treatment," *Pediatric Annals* (Vol. 13, no. 4, 1984) p. 300.

51 D. Cohen, W. Johnson, and M. Bowers, "Biogenic amines in autistic and atypical children: cerebrospinal fluid measure of homovanillica acid and 5-hydroxyindoleacetic acid," *Archives of General Psychiatry* (Vol. 31, no. 6, 1974) pp. 845-853.

52 Richard North, "Straight from the horse's mouth," *Nature* (January/February, 1985) p. 26.

53 Jack Cooper, Floyd Bloom and Robert Roth, *The Biochemical Basis of Neuropharmacology* 6th Edition (New York: Oxford University Press 1991) p. 408.

54 Christopher Gilberg, "The role of the endogenous opiods in autism and possible relationships to clinical features," in *Aspects of Autism: Biological Research*, Lorna Wing, ed. (Oxford: Alden Press, 1987) pp. 34-35.

55 Christopher Gilberg, "Treatment of Epilepsy in Autism" *Journal of Autism and Developmental Disorders* (Vol. 21, no. 1, 1991) pp. 61-77.

56 S.J. Hutt, C. Hutt and C. Ounstead, "A behavioral and electroencephalographic study of autistic children," *Journal of Psychiatric Research* (Vol. 3, 1965) p. 181-197.

57 J.P. Kootz, B. Marinelli and D. Cohen, "Modulation of response to environmental stimulation in autistic children," *Journal of Autism and Developmental Disorders* (Vol. 12, no. 2, 1982) p. 188.

58 Judith Rumsey, Ranjan Duara, Cheryl Grady, Judith Rapoport, Richard Margolin, Stanley Rapoport and Neal Cutler, "Brain metabolism in autism: resting cerebral glucose utilization rates as measured with positron emission tomography," *Archives of General Psychiatry* (Vol. 42, no. 5, 1986) pp. 452-453.

59 Z. Lipowski, "Sensory information inputs overload: behavioral effects," *Comprehensive Psychiatry* (Vol. 16, no. 3, 1975).

60 Z. Lipowsli, pp. 205 & 210-211.

61 Z. Lipowski, p. 211.

62 Steve Schwade, "Shedding light on sensitive hearing" *Prevention* (August, 1995) p.90.

63 Vernie McGee, "Feature letter" *Hyperacusis Network* (March, 1996) pp. 16-17.

64 John F. Kelly, "Feature letter" *Hyperacusis Network* (December, 1995) p. 18.

65 Nancy Carroll, "Feature letter" Hyperacusis Network (December, 1995)

66 H. Eysenck & M. Eysenck, *Personality and Individual Differences in a Natural Science Approach* (New York: Plenum Press, 1985) pp. 283-284.

67 J. Kagan, S. Reznick, N. Snidman, J. Gibbons & M. Johnson "Childhood derivatives of inhibition and lack of inhibition to the unfamiliar" *Child Development* (Vol. 59, 1988) pp. 1580-1589.

68 Z. Lipowski, p. 206.

69 Thanks to Dr. James Park of Edmonton, Alberta for initially suggesting this idea.

70 Judy Barron and Sean Barron, *There's a Boy in Here* (New York: Simon and Schuster, 1992), p. 83.

71 Annabel Stehli, p. 186.

72 Thomas McKean, "An alternate look at autistic perceptions" in *Proceedings from Autism: World of Options Conference* (Toronto: American Society of America and Autism Society Canada, July, 1993) pp. 29.

73 Judy Barron and Sean Barron, p. 227.

74 Judy Barron and Sean Barron, p. 229.

75 Judy Barron and Sean Barron, p. 118.

76 B. B. White & M. S. White, "Autism from the inside," *Medical Hypothesis* (Vol. 24, 1987) pp. 223-229.

Chapter Two

Mannerisms

Mannerisms are the abnormal patterns of behaviour displayed by individuals with autism. They range from extreme rigidity to running around in a continuous circular pattern. A variety of words are used to describe these behaviours: stereotypic, self-stimulating, bizarre, peculiar, abnormal or repetitive. Regardless of which term we use, these mannerisms all signify one factor - agitation resulting from the inability of the person with autism to deal with the stimulation of the environment in a normal manner.

For the caregiver, recognition that the behaviours are associated with the environment of the child is of prime importance. In order to help these children, we must take the time to observe their behaviours and connect them to what is happening with the environment, rather than accept that they occur for no discernible reason. For example, extreme reactions may be provoked by what we regard as trivial stimulus. A child may suddenly tense up, begin digging his nails into his flesh and scream, rear back into his chair and then bite his arm when a caregiver holds out her arms for a hug.[77] This extreme reaction begins to make sense if one takes into consideration acute tactile sensitivity. The arms of the nurse become a "threat" and the child reacts accordingly. His behaviour is definitely a form of protection.

Studies directly focused on the stereotyped movements of children with autism have found that these behaviours occur significantly more frequently with an increase in the complexity of the environment.[78] An increase in the frequency has also been noted in the presence of strangers, in new environments, or when a novel object is introduced into a familiar environment. These situations result in an increase in physiological arousal and thus appear to be associated with high levels of arousal, tension, and anxiety.[79] The intensity of stereotypical behaviours also increased following an encounter of a mildly aggressive nature.[80]

One our greatest difficulties may be an awareness of the level of intensity the individual with autism is experiencing, as compared to our own. A video of a young man and his staff member walking down the road showed him suddenly beginning to flap his hands. A short time later, a car passed. To a person with a normal range of hearing, the passing vehicle is usual and hardly worth noting. The man with autism, with his heightened auditory sense, noted the sound from a distance and began to protect himself from the noise, long before the vehicle arrived.

As the car passed it appeared this young man was deaf. The response to the direct sound of the car passing was ignored. In order to protect themselves from the onslaught of stimulation in the environment, those who have autism use repetitive behaviours to build up endorphins, which block out sensory stimulation. They appear to be deaf because their bodies have cut off all sensation to sound.

This lack of response has nothing to do with their capability to respond. It is the direct result of the use of repetitive behaviours or of the intense concentration by the individual on certain stimuli. Temple Grandin describes the effect of spinning coins and lids in the animated film *A is for Autism*: "I was intensely preoccupied with the movement of the spinning coin or lid and I saw nothing or heard nothing. I did it because it shut out sound that hurt my ears. No sound intruded on my fixation. It was like being deaf. Even a sudden noise didn't startle me out of my world."[81]

Scan Barron described his fascination with the call letters of radio and television stations. He would use the repetition of these letters in his mind to shut out people and his environment.[82]

This sensory reaction is not peculiar to individuals with autism. Sallie Bingham tells her life story in the autobiography *Passion and Prejudice, A Family Memoir*. Frustrated and hurt by the constant, cruel teasing of her older brother Worth, Sallie finally developed a method of protection.

On a car trip when she was eight or nine they passed a gasoline station just as he started to ridicule her. She began to repeat "gasoline station" to herself, over and over again and found that it totally blotted out his barbs. From then on, she was able to withdraw whenever she wanted to by repeating the words "gasoline station." It was an impenetrable defence, maddening to attackers.[83]

Since individuals with autism spend so much of their time protecting themselves from the onslaught of their environments, people do not take the time to recognize that the lack of response indicates a super sensitivity to stimuli and often dwell on the opposite. This is best represented in the book,[84] *The Ultimate Stranger, The Autistic Child* by Carl Delacato, in which a treatment based on hypo sensitivity (or lack of sensitivity) is described. It is also indicated by the prescription of eyeglasses and hearing aids by medical practitioners for many of the autistic population.

The syndrome of autism becomes totally confusing as definitions outline unusual reaction to perceptual stimuli, such as seeming to not hear certain sounds, yet overreacting to others. We must get past this problem and consider precisely what those who have autism are saying. They do realize they are involved in turning off their sensory systems. They do recognize there is a connection between being over stimulated and then having feelings that are "dead".[85] It is impossible to be physically deaf and hear sounds beyond the normal range of hearing at the same time. But it is not impossible for the brain to be creating this response by biochemical means.

The Role of Endorphins

As we mentioned in Chapter One, endorphins are one of the biochemicals produced in the brain. Endorphins are created as the natural response of the body to counteract pain and anxiety. When in pain or under stress, individuals with autism use repetitive behaviours to produce endorphins. A lack of response to stimulation, demonstrated by those who have autism, can be tied directly to the amount of endorphins that they have produced through the use of repetitive behaviours.

Individuals with autism have been measured to have higher levels of endorphins in their cerebrospinal fluid than normal subjects.[86] They are also known to suffer epileptic seizures,[87] which may well tie in with the response to these endorphins in the hippocampus of their brain. In his paper on the treatment of epilepsy in autism, Dr. Christopher Gilberg advises that a calm, well-structured environment for people with autism is often more important than the introduction of new or extra antiepileptic drugs.[88]

Too much stimuli coming in to the receptors of the brain will overload the response system, turning it off.[89] People with autism often purposely overload on stimulation to produce this effect. They may stare directly into a bright light, listen to extremely loud music or take part in self-mutilation by head banging, biting or pinching themselves.

One young man has explained that it is physically impossible for him to carry out his chore of vacuuming the floors until he has had time for "the sound to leave."[90] The sound of the vacuum cleaner is too stimulating for this young man to allow him to concentrate on the task. Once his body has built-up enough endorphins to cut off the sound, the job can be accomplished. Although a caring staff will allow extra time for this young man to complete his chores, we must also be aware that the sensory system has been temporarily cut off, and the person becomes lost in his own world. If we want those who have autism to learn and be part of our society, overloading the sensory system must be limited.

Cutting off sensation through the production of endorphins may seem like a simple and useful method of coping with stimulus sensitivity. However, once the endorphins are activated, reaction to all sensation is limited. The individual has a hard time reacting to any sensation, including those that are very important for bodily function. They will not be able to realize when they are hungry, or need to urinate, or have a bowel movement. Thus, it is extremely important to keep the level of endorphins as low as possible in order for the person to take part in day-to-day activities.

Individuals With Autism Say ...

> Whatever the reasons, I, as an autistic person, reacted in a fixated behaviour pattern in order to reduce arousal to my over stimulated nervous system.[91]

> The problem of perception confuses and haunts me. Colour and light bring intense pleasure, though they do not always make sense as simple vision. A greater quietude is gained from the self-stimulation I do, like forever flicking my hand or looking from the side with my eyes half closed. Jeffery Powell Jr.[92]

> There were two choices in coping with the nerve problem: I could retreat into my inner world and minimize the stimulation or I could fight fire with fire - find the most stimulating activity and "go for it". I remembered how the over stimulation from the carnival Rotor ride had helped to relieve my nerves. The ride's intense overpowering form of tactile and vestibular stimulation superseded my tendency to avoid vestibular and tactile stimulation. There was absolutely no way I could resist. Afterwards I had felt peace within for a brief time.[93]

> To fight boredom I resorted to my dream talk conversations. Sometimes I just sat by myself and rocked back and forth. Or I stared at my fingers; I found it helped me to turn off my busy mind so that I would not have to think about how bored I was. At other times I would spit on my finger and hold it up to the window, because by doing that, I could see all sorts of pretty colours as sunlight shone through the spit. I'm sure everyone thought I was behaving like a mindless idiot, but to me it was a form of amusement. Ian Whetherbee[94]

General Observations - Mannerisms That Indicate Agitation

Agitation is shown by the individual with autism in many different forms, which can be generally classified as abnormal repetitive behaviour. These behaviours may include pacing, rocking, flapping hands, arms or objects, staring into a bright light, screaming loudly, drinking Tabasco sauce straight from the bottle, spinning objects or self, chanting, humming, repeating an action over and over again such as closing a door or turning a light off and on, repeating a word or phrase over and over again. Self-injurious behaviours may include head banging, biting oneself, or pinching and picking at one's skin. Other, more serious, behaviours include aggression to others and destruction of objects in one's environment. The resources of each individual only limit the number of possible mannerisms.

There are various forms of stimulation from the environment, which affect people with autism that lead directly to the use of these mannerisms. Assessment of the situation is critical in determining just why a person is reacting as he is. Behaviours are used to block out direct over stimulation from many sources: the environment, a painful medical condition, stress due to trying to live up to the expectations of others, over stimulation from within due to a heightened emotional state (whether it be happiness, sadness, excitement or fear, the intuitive reaction to the emotional state of caregivers, or boredom).

Watch for the ability to complete a job or activity in the morning, but not in the evening. This is probably due to the build-up of one or more biochemicals in the body throughout the day's activities. Therefore, it is important to plan each day accordingly. Learning experiences and chores are best scheduled for the early morning, while relaxation and physical exercise may make better use of later hours.

The build-up of endorphins throughout the day may cause other problems. Children who suffer accidents in the evening may not show any pain. Darren White fell off a windowsill and broke his collarbone one evening. He showed no ill effects at the time and was sent to bed as usual. The next morning the pain was severe, and the full extent of his injuries were finally realized.[95]

Method of Care

The repetitive behaviours all link directly to stress in the environment. They signal AGITATION and must be recognized as such.

These behaviours can occur alone or be linked into a pattern. For example, pacing leads to flapping, which may lead to crying, which could lead to head banging, and so on. In these circumstances, it is possible to respond to the agitation long before a serious behaviour such as head banging ever occurs. On the other hand, an overwhelmingly painful situation can cause an individual with autism to head bang with no forewarning behaviours.

The repetitive behaviours must be eliminated, or at least controlled, because they cause the production of endorphins. It may be a relief to have the pain eliminated, but the presence of the endorphins also means that the individual loses the ability to respond to any stimulation. Without stimulation, our world becomes meaningless to them. They are not able to learn and develop as needed or to even be aware of what is going on around them. They are indeed lost in their own world.

Elimination of these behaviours occurs by focusing on the *reasons behind the behaviour* -- the over stimulation of the senses -- rather than on the behaviour itself. It is always very important to be aware of the stimulation in the environment and to modify the environment where needed. It is also crucial to communicate a recognition of the person's feelings and involvement at all times.

Pay close attention to your own emotional state when you are with people with autism. They have an uncanny ability to pick up your feelings, and to react to them as if they were their own. If you are feeling nervous, angry or frustrated, never try to hide your feelings from the person with autism, as they are going to be able to feel them anyway. Always remember that the calmer you are in any situation, the more relaxed they will be.

Life is not always calm and there are times you will have feelings that get in the way of being calm. During those times, get your feelings out in the open. Share with the person with autism that you are upset and that is has nothing to do with them. Once these feelings are out in the open, they are easier to cope with.

Physical exercise such as jogging builds up a reservoir of natural endorphins that also protect the individual but do not cut out the sensory response. Exercise can be used on a daily basis for preventative measures. It may also be used during bouts of agitation to help calm a person with autism. It can be used as a reward when a child has carried out a task well. Exercise can also be used to develop appropriate social responses. It is far better to jump on a trampoline, than on the furniture.

In the case of severe agitation, in which the cause cannot be identified, and where protection of the client is imperative, repetitive behaviours such as pacing or rocking can be used to calm the client for limited periods of time.

Behaviour modification techniques which focus on rewarding the absence of abnormal behaviour will likely result in the decrease of the specific behaviour, if one is using an effective reward.[96] However, it may also mean that these individuals will have to develop new behaviours to protect themselves from environmental stress. Since another undesirable behaviour may be added to the individual's repertoire, these techniques can become a waste of time and effort.

Agitation can be calmed effectively by using:

1. Soft, fleeting strokes on the bare skin; (the forearm is best) or a back massage for those who are not so tactile sensitive

2. A soft, calm voice with caring statements

3. Soft music (classical seems to work the best)

4. Time out in an empty, quiet, dimly lit space

5. Protein snacks

6. Physical exercise

7. Repetitive behaviours such as pacing or walking

8. vestibular stimulation such as swinging or rocking

While working with one young man who was relatively calm most of the time, we experienced him suddenly head banging against a wall, running wildly, and slapping himself. This behaviour was totally out of character for this client, who was usually rigid when under stress. We had no idea at all what was going on with him, but felt the severe behaviours indicated a serious problem.

As we studied the situation, we locked our arms around him and paced back and forth across the house, calming him sufficiently to be able to get him dressed and to a doctor.

Strep throat was diagnosed and medication was administered. In this way, we used one mannerism to allow him to build the endorphins that he needed, while protecting him from the more severe behaviours of head banging and slapping. Pacing was a far more acceptable choice at the time.

Medical problems can often lead to agitation and repetitive behaviours. A lack of communication compounds the problem. The theory that those who have autism do not experience pain in the same way we do, confuses the situation. The use of head banging has been described by one young man as "a way to let the pain out."[97] If we realize that this is what the person is attempting to do, we can then try to pinpoint the cause of the pain.

Earaches are often a recurring problem for most people with autism. Anyone who has suffered an earache can testify to the extent of pain as well as the desire to do anything to make it go away. Through careful monitoring of the behaviour of one young man, we discovered, that although the earache initially resulted in agitation and slapping of the head, it did not cause head banging. However, five minutes after antibiotic medication in a tablet form was administered, extreme head banging episodes occurred. In the past we had also observed this reaction shortly after generic forms of Ativan were administered. By comparing these two episodes, we concluded that the filler in the pills could be causing the problem and changed to a liquid form of the antibiotic whenever the client had an earache. This eliminated all head banging behaviour. Since that time, I have talked to many people who feel they have worked with people who are negatively reacting to antibiotic medication. It is imperative to consider that there may be negative reactions to different forms of medication and to monitor all situations very carefully.

It is also important to take medical problems into consideration when a person is engaged in severe forms of head banging. Headaches or toothaches are examples of medical conditions that may directly lead to the urge to "let the pain out."

Changes in the Environment

The bizarre behaviours of a person with autism are symptoms of the problem and not the problem itself. They are either a call for help or a method of protection. Delays in development occur when stimulation is blocked and learning does not occur. By concentrating on the sensory problems and creating a safe environment for the children, a caregiver may be able to eliminate the need for these behaviours.

Several studies, in which children with autism were placed in relative sensory isolation for long periods of time, have been carried out by different researchers. In England, two children were placed in a quiet room for 3-4 days (windowless, sound-proofed, and ventilated by air ducts and an exhaust fan) and then moved to a transition room (similar but with a window, and not sound-proofed) for the rest of the week, for a period of 6 weeks and a year. In both cases, stereotyped behaviours gradually decreased. Also observed was an increase in the use of visual and auditory responses, as well as normal play behaviour and initiation of physical contact with the caretakers.[98] Another interesting observation with both these children was their lack of awareness to stimulation before treatment. After treatment "they actively excluded sensory input - they covered their ears or tightly screwed up their eyes."[99]

A five-year old child, Jon, was confined to an experimental room in a Clinical Research Centre for a period of 74 days. All furnishings except a mattress were removed from the room and the lights were turned down. After eight days of isolation, gradual stimulation with people and objects was started. In the beginning, Jon appeared anxious, pacing, whirling, mumbling, and laughing to himself. As time passed, his "stereotypies" disappeared and he became playful with his caretakers, verbalized for food and drink, made good eye contact, and initiated physical contact with both the staff and his parents.[100]

One need not go to such an extreme to reduce agitation and stereotyped behaviours. Increases in classroom attention and task attention were noted in a study where only the levels of auditory input were reduced.[101] Self-stimulation, inappropriate behaviour, and inactivity were reduced in a classroom situation while redesigning the environment increased on-task behaviour. All decorations were removed, and walls and furniture were made one colour. The teacher wore dresses of the same colour and went without a watch or any jewellery or ornament.[102]

Facing a child towards the wall away from windows and doors and keeping desks clear of any materials not being used for the present task is recommended for effective classroom situations for children with autism at the Benhaven School.[103] Teacher Amy Lettick also cautions the use of various distractions such as long hair, bright colourful clothing, or jewellery while teaching.

At times, even moderate changes in our environment may be too difficult to organize. Children with autism may be expected to fit into a regular situation, especially during these times of integration or mainstreaming. One teacher told of an experience with her student in a kindergarten class.[104] Their classroom was in a separate building and any situation, especially during the cold winter months, had to be dealt with right in the midst of the other children. One day, the boy with autism was so agitated that no intervention on an individual level seemed to help. The teachers chose to respond by involving the whole classroom. They turned off all the lights, put on soft music, and had everyone lie quietly on the floor to enable this child to calm down. In the quiet darkness, his agitation gradually decreased. The kindergarten class could resume its normal activities. Two invaluable lessons were learned that day: the other children shared feelings other than their own, and the student with autism was given a special gift. His feelings were important enough for the whole class to take into consideration.

What is considered a safe environment? Throughout the following chapters, environmental suggestions will be offered to solve problems involved with the different senses. As a whole, we must consider safe environments those that do not over stimulate any sense. Keep decorations, such as pictures and ornaments, to a minimum. Colours should be soft and neutral (green seems to be a favourite). Noise levels can be lowered by the effective use of carpeting and drapery. Lighting should be indirect and soft. The perfect atmosphere should bring to mind the words "tranquillity" and "serenity" as one enters the room.

If it is not possible to offer individuals with autism this type of space, one should provide a totally empty area for them to use and give them the opportunity to relax and get themselves back on track. This area would not necessarily have to be big, but it should be soundproof, dim, and empty.

In strange or novel situations, any small room away from the rest of the group may provide a safe retreat. For example, while I was baby-sitting a group of children with autism, I used the bathroom as a retreat for one young lad who was overwhelmed by the whole situation. Once calm, he chose to spend most of his time in the coatroom away from the other children, away from all the toys, and away from all the activity. Since he was at a day care centre so his parents could take part in a support group, it was more sensible to allow the child a free choice for the time period, instead of forcing him to take part in-group activities.

Social Effects of Stereotyped Behaviours

Elimination of stereotyped behaviours is very important for two reasons. First, the blockage of stimulation that happens during these behaviours means that the individuals miss out on much of what they are supposed to be learning. Secondly, we must also be very aware of the social consequences of the behaviours. These behaviours are the greatest indication that the individual with autism is different from his peers. Studies have shown that subjects perceive people who display stereotyped behaviour, whether it is seen in a university student or in a mentally handicapped person, more negatively than people who do not display such behaviour.[105] In this study, there was a tendency for males to be more negative than females towards persons displaying stereotyped behaviours, and even more negative to those who were believed to be mentally handicapped. Socialization of the individual with autism in our "normal" society means that the perceptions of others are going to be very important. In order to protect those who have autism so they can be free to socialize without these detrimental effects, it is imperative to provide environments that are free from over stimulation.

Drugs and Aversives

It is important to be aware of the role of endorphins when measuring the effects of certain drugs on the autistic population. Naloxone/naltrexone are drugs, which counter the effects of the natural endorphins produced by the brain. They have been used to eliminate stereotyped behaviour in animals[106] and are being administered to people with autism.[107] Improvements in responsiveness, language, and stereotypic behaviours have been found in different studies,[108] sometimes combined with an increase in aggression and anxiety in each subject. Although these drugs may appear to make the caretaker's life easier and produce "results", which can be measured, they often remove the only protection the individual with autism may have from the stress of his environment. Creating more anxiety for those who have autism aggravates the problem, rather than alleviating it.

Another so-called cure for eliminating repetitive behaviours, especially those that are extreme, is the electric shock stick, which is used to force the individual to comply.[109] For those who are repulsed by the use of "cattle prods" in supposed medical treatment, the device is now called "SIBIS", a shorten form of "self-injurious behaviour inhibiting system." Advocates claim use is necessary for behaviours that cannot be controlled in any other manner.

The people who defend the use of these shock sticks claim that they are far less dangerous than allowing children to injure themselves or injure someone else.[110] They also claim electric shock is safer than drugs. These arguments are very valid to anyone who believes that the behaviour of the individual with autism occurs "for no reason". When you discover the reasons for the behaviours, the arguments for the use of electric shock become patently foolish. Why would we force a person to endure pain, for trying to avoid pain? It is far more logical and ethical to work on eliminating the cause of the behaviour.

Of course, electric shock is temporarily effective. Since the avoidance of pain is the total aim of the individual with autism, they will respond to avoid the electric shock. The abnormal behaviours that the caregivers want eliminated will disappear with the addition of more pain. The results can be measured and recorded. The question remains: how ethical and effective is it?

The use of aversives to eliminate undesirable behaviour was researched in the late sixties by Dr. O. Ivar Lovaas at the University of Southern California. His work with the autistic population has become well known throughout the world and films of his methods

are still used as teaching tools in the psychology departments of many universities. As Dr. Loaves continued this work, he discovered that although one second of mild shock on the arm would cause the client to stop undesirable behaviour, shock was not an effective tool to use over the long term. It was only effective as a temporary suppression. In most cases, the behaviours resumed unless one continued not only to administer shock, but also to escalate the shock level. Dr. Loaves currently cautions "you have to be super-cautious if you are going to use aversives. Super-cautious."[111]

Another aversive developed to use on people with autism was the administration of a puff of ammonia into the nose of the client. Ammonia is disturbing to us who have a normal level of smell. How much more agitating is it to those who are supersensitive to odour? When we take the sensory abilities of those who have autism into account, it becomes very apparent that the administration of ammonia is not only painful but can be described as an extreme form of torture and should never be allowed.

77 Corrine Hutt and S.J. Hutt, "Stereotypies and their relation to arousal: a study of autistic children," *Behavior Studies in Psychiatry* (Oxford: Pergamon Press, 1970) p. 193.

78 Corrine Hutt and S.J. Hutt, p. 190.

79 Corrine Hutt and S.J. Hutt, p. 192.

80 Corrine Hutt and S.J. Hutt, p. 189.

81 Dick Arnall (producer) and Tim Webb (director), *A is for Autism* [film] (London: A Finetake Production for Channel 4, 1992).

82 Judy Barron and Sean Barron, *There's a Boy in Here* (New York: Simon and Schuster, 1992), p. 120.

83 Sallie Bingham, *Passion and Prejudice a Family Memoir* (New York: Alfred A. Knopf, 1989) p. 19.

84 Carl H. Delacato, *The Ultimate Stranger The Autistic Child* (Novato, California: Academic Therapy Publications, 1974) update.

85 "Journey into an autistic mind of a "high functioning" autistic young lady, aged 26 years," *The International Autistic Research Organization Newsletter* (January, 1991) p. 5.

86 Christopher Gilberg, "The role of the endogenous opiods in autism and possible relationships to clinical features," in *Aspects of Autism: Biological Research*, Lorna Wing, ed. (Oxford: Alden Press, 1987) pp. 34-35.

87 Christopher Gilberg, "The role of the endogenous opiods in autism and possible relationships to clinical features," in *Aspects of Autism: Biological Research*, Lorna Wing, ed. (Oxford: Alden Press, 1987) pp. 34-35.

88 Christopher Gilberg, p. 74.

89 Masel Mesulam, *Principles of Behavioral Neurology* (Philadelphia: F.A. Davis Company, 1985) p. 332.

90 Barbara Barker, "Looking at behavior from a different perspective," *Hands Reaching Hands* [newsletter] (Toronto: The Metro Toronto Chapter, Autism Society Ontario, April, 1993) p. 3.

91 Temple Grandin and Margaret Scariano, *Emergence: Labeled Autistic* (Novato, California: Arena Press) p.74.

92 Jeffrey Powell Jr., "Writing workshop" handout, *Living with the Questions Facilitated Conference* (Syracuse, New York, May 1996) p. 8.

93 Temple Grandin and Margaret Scariano, p. 89.

94 Ian Wetherbee, "M-Y...N-A-M-E...I-S...I-A-N" *Guideposts, a Practical Guide to Successful Living* (August, 1993) p. 5.

95 B.B. White and M.S. White, " "Autism from the inside," *Medical Hypotheses* (Vol. 24, 1987) p. 225.

96 O.I. Lovaas, "Behavioral treatment and normal educational and intellectual functioning in young autistic children," *Journal of Consulting and Clinical Psychology* (Vol. 55, 1987) pp. 3-9.

97 Karl Evans, personal communication from his mother, used with permission.

98 G. Stroh & D. Buick, "The effect of relative sensory isolation on the behavior of two autistic children," in *Behavior Studies in Psychiatry*, C. Hutt & S.J. Hutt (eds). (Oxford: Pergamon Press, 1970) pp. 161-173.

99 G. Stroh and D. Buick, p. 171.

100 William Maier, "Sensory deprivation therapy of an autistic boy," *American Journal of Psychotherapy* (Vol. 25, 1970) p. 228-245.

101 Joan Fassler & Dale Bryant, "Disturbed children under reduced auditory input: a pilot study," *Exceptional Children* (November, 1971) p. 203.

102 Pieter Duker & Eef Rasing, "Effects of designing the physical environment on self-stimulation and on-task behavior in three autistic-type developmentally disabled individuals," *Journal of Autism and Developmental Disorders* (Vol. 19, no. 3, 1989) p. 454.

103 Amy Lettick, "On structuring a Lesson," *Journal of Learning Disabilities* (Vol. 6. no. 1, 1973) p. 12.

104 Panel Discussion: The Coice of Experience. Teachers who are Integrating. Autism Today Conference (Calgary, Alberta, 1994.

105 R. Jones, D. Wint, & N. Ellis, "The social effects of stereotyped behavior," *Journal of Mental Deficiency Research* (Vol. 34, 1990) p. 266.

106 Richard North, p. 26.

107 Tom Berney, "The Pharmacotherapy of Autism," *Experimental Biology and the Autistic Syndromes* (Durham: National Autistic Society and Sunderland Polytechnic, 1989) p. 7.

108 M. Campbell, J. Overall, A. Small, M. Sokol, E. Spencer, P. Adams, R. Foltz, K. Monti, R. Perry, M. Nobler, & E. Roberts, "Naltrexone in autistic children: an acute open dose range tolerance trial," *Journal of American Child and Adolescent Psychiatry* (Vol. 28, 1989) p. 204.

109 Thomas Linscheid, Brian Iwata, Robert Ricketts, Don Williams and James Griffen, "Clinical Evaluation of the Self-Injurious Behavior Inhibiting System (SIBIS)," *Journal of Applied Behavior Analysis* (Vo. 23, no.1, 1990) pp. 53-78.

110 Bernard Rimland, "Risks and benefits in the treatment of autistic children. A risk/benefit perspective on the use of aversives," *Journal of Autism and Childhood Schizophrenia* (Vol. 8, no. 1, 1978) p. 104.

111 Andrew Heyword & Susan Zirinsky (producers) and Don Ray King (director), "Shock Value", *Eye to Eye with Connie Chung* [television film] (CBS Inc, March 3, 1994).

Chapter Three

Tactile

Touch is the most important sense in the development of a social human being. It is usually the first sensory response recognized by the parents of children with autism, which indicates their child, is different. Some babies with autism rarely enjoy being held or cuddled and struggle for freedom in their parents' arms. As they grow older, they do not develop the behaviour of "assuming an anticipatory posture preparatory to being picked up", a major factor in Kanner's original description of this syndrome.[112] As with all areas of autism, individual differences must be taken into account.

Parents who recognize their babies' feelings adapt to their needs by leaving them alone, or letting them lie undisturbed in their cribs or playpens as much as possible. This attitude may have contributed to the definition of refrigerator parents in the fifties and sixties.[113] However, the parents' acceptance does not indicate coldness, but instead illustrates the empathy they feel for their child and the respect they have for their individual feelings. On the other side, the people who are unwilling, or unable, to recognize tactile defensive behaviour as a method of communication, forcefully hold the screaming, struggling child, causing extreme trauma.

If we take a close look at the normal development of an infant and parent relationship, it is easy to comprehend where tactile problems might cause confusion. What is the instinctive response of a mother who wants to comfort a crying baby? Holding and cuddling. So, we have a situation where a child in pain cries out, using the normal method of infant communication. The parent or other caregiver also reacts in the normal fashion by picking up and holding the child. This results in an added level of pain. The memories of the trauma caused by this early pain have been documented by Jeanne Simmons.[114]

Gordon, one of a group of young lads in a group home, was watching the movie "*A Child is Born*". As the actual birth was pictured on the screen, he panicked, jumping up on the table and gasping out his fear that the baby would get angry if the mother touched it. This story was included in this book to illustrate the ability of those who have autism to recall early memories. Could this memory be an indication of how early in life babies with autism react to the pain of touch, and how extreme this pain must be?

The infant with autism quickly realizes when his method of communication - crying - is not giving him the desired results. The young child is forced to develop new and unique methods of communicating feelings. Is it not better to remain silent than to cry out? If one is avoiding tactile stimulation, silence is an effective defence. Caregivers, including parents, usually do not rush to pick up a silent baby.

These new methods of communication will last a lifetime and will be extremely difficult to change. Expressing one's feelings out loud will provoke fear, while silence will provide protection. This limits the ability of the person with autism to express any feelings in any manner for the rest of his or her life.

When our tactile system is heightened, touch that is usually comforting and enjoyable becomes unbearable. This reaction is vividly described by individuals with autism. Furthermore, when one considers many of the behaviours used by the autistic population, one can readily see a connection between tactile sensitivity and behaviour. For example, is it not logical to tiptoe when one is walking if the soles of one's feet are especially sensitive? Walk across a gravel road in bare feet and watch your own natural reaction. It gives the tiptoe walk of the person with autism a new meaning very quickly.

While reading through descriptions of autistic behaviour, or case studies of individuals with autism, one is constantly presented with the idea that behaviour occurs for no discernible reason. For instance, in the textbook *Children in Need of Special Care*, Thomas Weihs describes a young boy with autism standing at a window, swishing the curtain in front of his face.[115] When approached by the author, who reaches over to place his hand on the lad's shoulder, the boy suddenly shrieks and throws himself on the bed, hiding under the bedclothes. The doctor goes on to describe the client's behaviour, finally coming to the conclusion that children with autism "are compelled to do things that fall out of the ordinary scope of motivation."[116]

One young lad was very upset when he was told that a male staff member would look him after for a weekend. When asked "why" by the supervisor he replied, "He hurts me".

The supervisor was instantly alert. She could not believe that the man in question was hurting those in his care, but she was also very attentive to the feelings of the youngster. "What do you mean?" she asked.

The little boy replied, "When you touch me you do this." He lightly ran his hand down the length of his arm. "And it feels good. But when he touches me, he does this." He held his hand on his shoulder, "And it hurts -- it feels like fire running through my body."

Closer examination of these two cases allows us to recognize certain similarities. Is not the little boy who screams and slips away from the grasp of the shoulder using body language instead of words to communicate the same message as the second boy? The repetitive swishing of the curtain reveals that this child is already agitated, though we have not been told the reason. Obviously, the therapist has the habit of grasping the shoulder and the child expects the pain to be overwhelming. His protective behaviour emerges.

Throughout the remainder of this chapter we will look at descriptions provided by individuals with autism that explain their reactions to the sense of touch. General behaviours to watch for that can be related directly back to tactile sensitivity will be outlined. Next, I will describe a method of care which, when used with a person with autism, will make an important difference in his or her life. Using these methods will help people with autism cope with excessive stimulation in their environments. Finally, these methods provide human touch that is pleasant and comforting, touch that will allow healthy social development.

Individuals with Autism Say ...

> "I was six months old when Mother noticed that I was no longer cuddly and that I stiffened up when she held me. When I was a few months older, Mother tried to gather me in her arms, and I clawed at her like a trapped animal." Temple Grandin[117]
>
> "I never used to like being picked up and cuddled. I screamed as though I was on a roller coaster if anyone tried to pick me up. I also hated it when my teacher, Mrs. Ingram, tried to make me hold my pencil properly or my parents tried to make me do up my laces or shirt buttons. They had no idea of what was wrong with me at the time. And, since I thought it happened to everyone, I didn't tell anyone. Nevertheless, I found such treatment

excruciating.... I don't like pressing my lips on spoons or glass hard either." Darren White[118]

"There were other things I had to do every day that made me quite uncomfortable as well. One of these was taking a bath. I felt acutely uncomfortable sitting upright in the bathtub, so I didn't enjoy taking a bath in the least. I absolutely hated the way my bottom felt against the tub, and I couldn't make myself think about something else so I wouldn't feel it. When I tried to sit normally it felt "squishy" and I was extremely sensitive to this feeling. I couldn't shake it off. It was the same feeling I used to have when I couldn't stand to touch our rugs with my bare feet. To make it more bearable, I shifted most of my weight onto one side so that only a part of me came into contact with the bathtub. When they insisted I "sit right" it only compounded the problem. I had no choice - I had to sit in an unnatural way so baths were a trying experience. Also it made me feel that there was something wrong with me because I had to sit that way." Sean Barron[119]

"The most terrifying and confusing of all is touch, which seems intense. Reality reappears as strident burning if my clothes are new or tight or the wrong fabric. When starting to facilitate, I had to weaken my response to being held by the hand and I often needed to get away from the intensity of all the simultaneous stimulation. I learned to accommodate the touch of familiar facilitators, but the need to escape situations explains why I sometimes walk away or make another self-created noise to focus myself." Jeffrey Powell Jr.[120]

Indications of Tactile Sensitivity

As caregivers we have to assume there is a reason for every behaviour that the individual with autism exhibits. It is our duty to assess the situation and try to discover why the behaviour is taking place. Specific areas to watch for tactile problems include:

- Rejection of human touch. This may include pushing or pulling away from, struggling, screaming or crying out, becoming stiff and tense, becoming very limp and passive, or the use of stereotypic behaviours such as flapping or reciting words while being touched.
- Rejection or discomfort at the touch of clothing. Watch especially for rough textures and restrictive clothing. Rough seams or labels at the neckline may be a problem. Changes in fabric or in types of clothing (going from long pants in the summer to shorts) may reveal discomfort. New clothing may be too starchy to wear.
- Sensitive feet. Walking on tiptoes or refusal to wear certain footwear, especially new shoes or boots, are the main indicators of this problem. Sean Barron describes his difficulty walking in bare feet as strange and awful.[121]
- Avoidance of games that involve tactile contact such as kicking or catching a ball.
- Discomfort when sitting in one place for any length of time.
- Genital manipulation or masturbation. This is commonly the sign of lack of quality tactile experiences.

- Sensitivity to extreme changes in temperature. Water at body temperature can become an obsession. Hot or cold water causes fear. Very hot weather causes agitation.

- The mouth is a very sensitive area. Watch for problems while eating. Going from a liquid diet to a solid one is usually very traumatic. Refusal to use utensils, certain cups or glasses, or try out new foods will occur. The temperature of food may be tested on the tongue or chin.

- The tips of the fingers are also very sensitive, so watch for problems holding things and doing tasks, especially where a firm grip is needed, such as doing up zippers or buttons, holding a fork or writing with a pencil.

- There also may be difficulty in writing neatly, or carrying out a task, which is neat enough to meet the expectations of others.

- There may be a great desire for cleanliness, a dislike for sticky or dirty hands.

Method of Care

Touch

Youth really needs
To be touched
The reason I do not know
I only feel it is
Perhaps
The quietest form
of growth
David Eastham[122]

As caregivers to individuals with autism, we have to shut down a natural human response - the impulse to touch those whom we are caring for. We must stop and realize, at all times, that the touch we deliver and enjoy may well be painful. We must stop and take the time to realize that our hugs do not feel the same to them. We must not, at any time, take their withdrawal personally. It is a means of protection for the person with autism, and we must respect it as such.

On the other hand, tactile stimulation, especially physical contact with another human being, is important to each and every one of us, including the person with autism. It is of prime importance to find a method of touch that is bearable to those who have autism.

There may be areas in this tactile section that seem to provide contradictory advice. Due to the problems with tactile sensitivity that lead to pain and the prerequisite of the human psyche to receive tactile stimulation, these contradictions form a considerable portion of the dilemma of working with those with autism. Definition of the situation is always critical to tactile stimulation in the care of those who have autism.

For example, many people with autism claim to have a constant low level pain running through their bodies, just under their skin, at all times.[123] This pain often drives them to distraction, so they are unable to concentrate on whatever else is going on around them. The pain can be eliminated through the use of deep pressure. Individuals with autism have created many ways to provide the deep pressure to themselves such as sleeping between mattresses instead of on them, rolling up in rugs and blankets, taking hard showers and wearing weighted vests or T-shirts that are one size too small. Temple Grandin's squeeze machine was developed to cope with this pain. People who are suffering from this pain will often withdraw from your touch, at the same time they are looking for deep pressure they can apply to themselves. The issue at stake is the need for control over the amount and kind of pressure that is applied.

One also has to be aware that people with extreme tactile sensitivity react differently than those people who have either matured to the point that touch is no longer a problem for them, or who are not as sensitive from the start. Thus, light touch for some people is comforting, while it drives others crazy. The only way to figure out which type of touch is effective for the person you are working with is to try them out and watch the response. Even if they are unable to tell you in words, their behaviour will quickly reveal whether the touch you are giving is good for them. My general rule of thumb is the lower functioning the person I am working with, the lighter the touch I use, until I get to know their individual preference.

Individuals with autism recognize the lack of touch when you initially approach them as genuine respect for their feelings. By not touching them, you allow them the freedom to realize that you do understand what they are experiencing. Resisting the urge to make physical contact allows the possibility of trust to occur in a much shorter period of time.

Only after you are certain that you have reached a level of trust with the individual do you touch a person with autism.

General Guidelines for Care

Never forcefully hold hands, arms, shoulders or any part of the body.

Never insist on hugs and kisses or use hugs and kisses as a system of reward. Always be aware that our hugs and kisses may very well not be comforting or even comfortable for the individual with autism. In contrast to our normal method of hugging, Sara Miller endorses what she calls the `Super Sensory Hug'.

> Approach from the front so you don't surprise them. Get behind them. From the back, do a `Bear hug' under their arms at a level or just below their rib cage. Firmly squeeze. WHISPER anything nice you want them to remember into their dominant ear, but turn your mouth away from their ear or neck so the air current from your breath doesn't interfere with the message.[124]

Many parents have told me that their son or daughter has always approached them backwards when asked for a hug. They never realized that the child was showing them how, like Sara, they preferred to be hugged.

According to Sara, kisses on the forehead are far more enjoyable than on the cheek, where they feel like steel wool scratching the skin.[125] Darren White demonstrated this behaviour as a very young child. Videos taken when his baby brother was first brought home from the hospital show Darren gently kissing the baby's forehead. Darren never touched his brother in any other way when he was young. If we take the time to watch closely how these children react to others, we may learn how they want to be treated by us. Watch how they kiss others, and respond to them in the same way.

Never hold any part of their body for any length of time. Donna Williams described her reaction to having a part of her body held as "the imprint of your touch stays in my skin for two to three hours".[126]

If you have to touch them, use soft caressing strokes on the arm. This calming behaviour by a child with autism was demonstrated by Raun Kaufman when he was very young. Another little boy in a playground was frightened and began to cry. Raun moved cautiously towards him and stroked his arm softly until the child stopped crying.[127] If they pull away from this type of touch, it is likely too light for them. If so, massage their backs or arms with strong, deep strokes instead of light ones. Keep your hands moving.

Don't hover over them. Give them space!

Don't insist on shaking hands in greeting. "High fives" are more comfortable for them, but not as acceptable once they become adults. Just a wave or a spoken hello will do.

Wrestling and tickling type games seem to be acceptable. These activities provide strong tactile stimulation, but never grasp one part of the body for any length of time. When indulging in this activity remember to watch the reactions of the individual with autism closely. They will tell us if it is too much by their reaction.

Provide soft, loose fitting clothing. Do not vary the type of material and style from one outfit to another. Watch for sharp seams, (French seams are the best), constricting or sharp collars, and always cut any labels out of the necklines. Temple Grandin claims that it takes her body up to two weeks to adjust to a change in clothing, whether in style (from slacks to skirts) or in fabric. She copes with this problem by always choosing to dress the same.[128]

Always wash new clothes a couple of times before the individual with autism wears them to eliminate the starch which is added to make the clothes look crisp and new in the store. The more clothes have been washed, the better they will feel to the individual with autism. Be aware that the detergents you use may also cause difficulties.

However, there are materials that become more scratchy and unbearable, the more they are washed.[129] This condition is often found in cotton blend fabrics. A favourite item of clothing may suddenly begin to cause problems and be rejected by the individual with autism. If so, respect these feelings.

Straps on helmets and hats must not be too restrictive, as one cannot concentrate on the activity if there is too much pressure on any part of the body. The extreme result of a reaction to clothing is illustrated by one incident in the life of Temple Grandin.[130] One day, her mother insisted that she keep her hat on as they were driving down the road. Temple found this hat to be too tight and uncomfortable, so in desperation she threw it out the window. The result of her mother's reaction was a traffic accident.

Comfortable socks and shoes are a must. Mark gave up walking on his toes when he was given a pair of moccasins with rabbit fur lining. He also started to refuse to go out of the house and threw his shoes in the garbage. This was described as bizarre behaviour until one realized that he was forced to change out of his slippers whenever he left the house. If persons with autism refuse to wear a particular pair of shoes, instead of insisting, respect their wishes. The shoes may hurt in ways of which you are not aware.

Sara Miller warns against knee socks and sports socks, which are tight against the calf muscles.[131] She finds the scrunchy type of socks the most comfortable. She also is uncomfortable with socks that have absorbent terry soles on the inside as they irritate her feet. She chooses to wear them inside out.

Never insist that individuals with autism sit in one place for long periods of time. Let them move about during the day, perhaps standing for some tasks and sitting for others. If the task requires sitting for long periods of time take short breaks to walk around for a while to relax the skin areas. On long drives, respect the need for movement and allow a break now and then to run off some energy and to relax the tactile pressure. Be aware that seat belts in cars may be too restrictive and lead to agitation.

Genital manipulation is a pleasure-seeking behaviour. With a program of other touch that is pleasant, instead of painful, this behaviour should fade on its own.[132]

Water is very pleasurable for some people with autism if the temperature is not extreme. Bathing, swimming, and water play can be used for times of relaxation and to calm agitation. For others, bathing may be uncomfortable. Rough towels may cause problems. Be aware that all problems around water may not relate to the tactile area. Hearing and smell may also be affected, so keep an open mind.

Do not insist that those who have autism hold pencils, eating utensils and so on in the "proper" manner. A palm grip causes less stress than using the tips of the fingers. If there is refusal to use writing tools, it may be more advantageous to go to other means such as the computer for the written word. As time passes and the tactile system matures, this sensitivity decreases. They adjust to the most comfortable method of using these tools on their own which is usually the "proper" method. Also, there are foam triangles available to put on pencils to make them softer, which may make a difference in the ability to write

Many with autism will choose to adapt to our methods if they have been allowed to learn to eat and write in their own way first. Others may insist on using their own methods throughout their lives. An illustrated view of unique eating methods, developed by the autistic individual to protect himself from pain, can be seen on the movie *Rainman* where Raymond uses a toothpick instead of a fork to eat.[133]. Being aware that tasks may cause pain will make a big difference in your frustration while working with people with autism.

For example, one young child had difficulty in zipping up his jacket. As we were leaving for day care, his mother asked him to zip it up. He struggled with the zipper. Unable to get the zipper started, he gave a piercing scream. His mother did the zipper up. Earlier, I had seen him working with various zippers on a toy snake. It was evident that he not only knew what they were for, but also how to operate them. While sharing this information with his parents, I mentioned that his jacket zipper was very difficult for this boy, and that it was likely causing him a lot of pain when he attempted to do it up. He was playing in a nearby corner and he turned and looked at me and said "It is very hard, Gail."

Since this child does know how to put a zipper together and the stress on the tips of his fingers results in agitation, which in turn causes frustration for the caregivers as well as the child, I believe he should not be expected to zip this particular zipper. He should always be allowed to try, but if he does not succeed, accept it without fuss and do it for him. He is not doing up his zipper because it hurts, not because he is developmentally delayed or lazy. Once we accept the real reasons for this child's reaction to the jacket zipper, he no longer needs to get attention with a piercing scream. He is free to ask for help in another way.Life becomes much easier for everyone involved.

Texture may play a big part in the refusal to use something. For example, many individuals with autism insist on using only one glass to drink. This may relate to the texture of the glass, compared to others they have had contact with, which were found to be unbearable. The insistence on "sameness" is a definite attempt by individuals with autism to protect themselves from discomfort.

Hand-over-hand is a method of instruction used by many educators to teach tasks to individuals affected by autism, especially in the area of life skills. I have taught them different tasks related to the preparation and cleanup of meals using both hand-over-hand techniques and through my own method. I took the environment into account and then taught by imitation. In both instances, the task was taught and seemed to be learned. Using my method the tasks gradually became self-initiated and generalized to other environments. I believe there is a high level of stress in many of the sensory areas, especially tactile, caused by the use of hand-over-hand methods.

When developing leisure activities for people with autism, be creative in taking the tactile experience into account. For example, playing catch with a frisbee is preferable to using a hard ball. Inflatable balls are also easier for those who have autism to use. Games, which are based on keeping a beach ball or balloon up in the air, will likely produce a better response than soccer, where the ball must be kicked, or baseball, in which it must be hit.

Sheepskin, used as a covering for mattresses, chairs or even desks[134] has been found to be effective when working with autistic people.

A light physical touch or tap will often get individuals with autism moving again if they are “stuck” in a certain position or movement.[135]

Older autistic individuals may often crave much more physical contact than the rest of the autistic population.[136] It is important to be available to not only supply this contact, but to do it in a manner, which benefits the particular individual. If they can't tell you how much they need in words, watch their behaviours carefully and respond accordingly.

Massage is beneficial for people with autism if properly applied. For those who are extremely tactile sensitive light, soft massage can be used as a reward, to calm agitation and during periods of relaxation. Massage should be first tried on the forearm, as it is not as sensitive as other areas of the body.[137] When carrying out light massage, always use downward strokes that follow the direction of the nervous system from the brain to the outer ends of the body.[138] Many of the individuals with autism, who have managed to become active, self-sufficient members of society, had parents who recognized the need for soft massage in infancy and provided it. Through the use of light massage on the arms, a teenager’s response to physical contact progressed from passive resistance to hugs to cuddling into our chests as he squeezed tightly. In Sweden a light baby massage is recommended as a regular treatment in the area of autism and results are promising.[139]

On the other hand, deep massage is the touch of choice for people who find light touch uncomfortable. Again, it can be used to calm agitation, as a reward, and during periods of relaxation. I always begin with very light touch to discover how the person responds. If they flinch and pull away they are indicating they need deep pressure. Although the light touch is uncomfortable to those who prefer deep pressure, it does not hurt the individual as beginning with deep pressure on those who need light touch would do.

Regular deep massage is useful for most people with autism who are in their late teens and adult years, providing they have already learned to cope with physical touch. It provides the tactile stimulation, which their bodies have gone without for so many years and should be incorporated into any weekly schedule.

Vibration is used by individuals with autism to calm themselves or as a substitute for self-injurious behaviours, such as biting. Some people find their own sources of vibration and become fixated on electric motors or vacuum cleaners. Since the vibration causes a build up of endorphins and blocks out feelings, it is advised to be cautious and limit exposure to vibration when working with those who have autism.

Epsom salt baths on a regular basis provide relaxation, which can last for hours.

Self-mutilation has been described as the deep-seated need for tactile stimulation due to a damaged nervous system that limits tactile feeling.[140] This theory is directly opposite to the descriptions by individuals with autism, and the effects we have described in this book. It also contradicts claims by people who are not autistic and who self-mutilate.[141] As caregivers, we must realize that hurting oneself is not an attempt by the person to provide stimulation, but instead a method of creating endorphins in their bodies and therefore limiting the effect of incoming stimulation. By providing an environment where the stimulation is not overpowering, and providing tactile stimulation that is pleasurable instead of painful, self-mutilation will fade on its own.

Self-mutilation is an indication of a severe problem in the environment. If you are with someone who begins to self-mutilate, whether by biting, pinching or head banging, when they have never done so before, you must realize that this is an indication that they are suffering from something, whether it be a sensory stimulation problem, or an extreme reaction to a person they have to deal with on a regular basis. Self-mutilation works quickly in providing pain-killing endorphins and once people have learned to use it, sadly they often resort to choosing it first, as it relieves the pain so quickly. They also may learn to use it in order to produce a desired reaction from people around them. It is so much better to protect our little ones all the time so they never have to reach the point of choosing to partake in self-mutilation.

Individuals with autism enjoy deep pressure in which they are in control of the amount of pressure applied to themselves, such as burying under things to play, rolling up in a rug, or cuddling under a pile of blankets.[142] The key to pleasure is having control over the situation. They may also use deep pressure to calm themselves when agitated, such as falling full length on their front or back.

One deep pressure activity, which can be tried in a classroom as a game, is making peanut butter and jelly sandwiches. A mat is placed on the floor and represents the first slice of bread. The child with autism lies on the mat, becoming the peanut butter. Another "slice of bread" (mat) is placed on top of the child. A second child becomes the jelly. Another mat completes the `sandwich' or more layers can be added. This activity allows peers to help the child with autism cope with his situation in a fun way.

Temple Grandin has produced a `squeeze machine', which is now commercially available. This machine allows a person to be `hugged' or tightly squeezed in a manner in which the individual has complete control.[143]

Individuals with autism also enjoy the tactile pressure created by movement on a swing or when spun around, either by someone or on a machine like the rides found at a carnival. The extremes in tactile, auditory and odour at such places often push those who have autism to over stimulation, which, as we have already mentioned, allows them to feel good for a while.[144]

Occupational and physical therapists are beginning to be involved in this field, called sensory integration, as a specialty.[145] These specialists may provide more information as well as actual therapy and materials. The term they use in regards to touch is Tactile Defensiveness.

Be very cautious when you get involved in this therapy. There is a considerable difference in the attitude that one must "fix something that is broken" compared to one in which we provide methods of care which allow individuals to cope with their situation and become the best they can be. Other therapists concentrate on making the disabled person "normal". This attitude can again do much harm, as one then ignores the actual feelings and experiences of those we are trying to help. We also must be very aware of where the particular definition of "normal" has originated.

Conclusion

Human touch is extremely important for human growth and development. People, who have gone without physical human contact as infants, suffer severe developmental problems. Studies on premature babies, who spent months in incubators after their birth, indicate that a lack of tactile stimulation in infancy leads to problems in the areas of language skills, motor skills, toileting, emotional levels, anxiety and stress levels, and sensory acuity.[146] These all play an important role in the differences in development seen in children with autism. Because of these studies, programs of tactile contact are now part of the day-to-day life of incubator babies. All in all, it appears that the more touching you get as an infant and small child, the better off you are.

On the other hand, over stimulation through touch for people with autism leads to the need for protection from pain. This results in withdrawal and the necessity to develop "mannerisms" which build up endorphins to cope with the pain. It is imperative to find ways to touch individuals with autism that provide comfort and enjoyment. Pleasurable tactile stimulation will provide the opportunity for normal development.

112 Leo Kanner, "Autistic disturbances of affective contact," in *Classic Readings in Autism*, Anne Donnellan, ed. (New York: Teacher's College Press, 1985) p. 41.

113 Bruno Bettelheim, *The Empty Fortress Infantile Autism and the Birth of Self* (New York: The Free Press, 1972) p. 21-27.

114 Jeanne Simmons and Sabine Oishi, *The Hidden Child The Linwood Method for Reaching the Autistic Child* (Kensington Maryland: Woodbine House, 1987) p. 222.

115 Thomas J. Weihs, *Children in Need of Special Care: Human Horizons Series* (London: Souvenir Press, 1971) p. 74.

116 Thomas J. Weihs, p. 84

117 Temple Grandin and Margaret Scariano, *Emergence Labeled Autistic* (Novato, California: Arena Press, 1986) p. 19.

118 White, Darren, *More Autobiography* (unpublished manuscript).

119 Judy Barron and Sean Barron, *There's a Boy in Here* (New York: Simon and Schuster, 1992) p.96.

120 Jeffrey Powell, Jr., "Writing workshop" handout, *Living with the Questions Facilitated Conference* (Syracuse, New York, May 1996) p. 9.

121 Judy Barron and Sean Barron, *There's a Boy in Here* (New York: Simon and Schuster, 1992), p. 15.

122 David Eastham, *Understand* (Ottawa, Ontario: Oliver Pate, 1989) p. 32, used with permission.

123 Thomas McKean, speaking at the Autism '96 Conference sponsored by Future Horizons, Inc. in Denver, Colorado, September 1995, used with permission.

124 Sara Miller, " Does the Princess Have PDD? Different is good: it's back-to-school time," *Autism Society of Southeastern Wisconsin Newsletter* (September, 1993), used with permission.

125 Sara Miller.

126 Donna Williams, speaking at the Facilitated Communication Conference in Syracuse, New York, May 1995.

127 Barry Kaufman, *Son Rise* (New York: Warner Books, 1976) p. 126.

128 Temple Grandin, speaking at the National Autism Society Conference in Los Angeles, July 1990.

129 Sara Miller, "My personal autism spectrum theory" Does the Princess Have PDD? (unpublished manuscript, 1993).

130 Temple Grandin and Margaret Scariano, pp. 17-18.

131 Sara Miller, "Does the Princess Have PDD? Brushing techniques: sensory defensiveness," *Autism Society of Southeastern Wisconsin Newsletter* (March, 1993).

132 Ashley Montagu, *Touching The Human Significance of the Skin* Third Edition (New York: Harper & Row, Publisher, 1986) p. 224.

133 Peter Guber & Jon Peters (Producers) & Barry Levison (Director), *Rainman* [film] (Culver City, CA: MGM/UA Home Video, Inc, 1988).

134 Temple Grandin, "Teaching tips from a recovered autistic," *Focus on Autistic Behavior* (Vol. 3, no. 1, 1988) p. 4.

135 Barbara Barker, "Looking at behavior from a different perspective," *Hands Reaching Hands* (newsletter) (Toronto: The Metro Toronto Chapter, Autism Society Ontario, April, 1993) p. 3.

136 Thomas McKean, p. 30.

137 Donna Williams, *Nobody Nowhere* (Toronto, Doubleday Canada Limited, 1992) p. 217.

138 Patricia St. John, *The Secret Language of the Dolphins* (New York: Summit Books, 1991) p. 202.

139 Personal conversation with Inger Nilsson, Psychologist from Stockholm, Sweden.

140 Edward Carr, "The motivation of self-injurious behavior: a review of some hypotheses," in *Classic Readings in Autism*, Anne Donnellan, ed. (New York: Teachers College Press, 1985) p. 303.

141 Nick Supina, "Drawing out the pain," *Dialog* (Edmonton, Alberta Canada) p. 28.

142 Temple Grandin and Margaret Scariano, p. 33, and Thomas McKean, "An alternate look at autistic perceptions" in *World of Options* Conference proceedings (Toronto: Autism Society of America and Autism Society Canada, July 1993) pp. 29-30.

143 For more information on the squeeze machine and how to order contact: Therafin Corporation, P.O. Box 848, Mokena, IL 60448, (708) 479-1515 or (800) 843-7234.

144 Temple Grandin and Margaret Scariano, pp. 76 & 89.

145 For a book on this subject see Jean Ayres, *Sensory Integration and the Autistic Child* (Los Angeles: Western Psychological Services, 1979). The Ayres Clinic in Los Angeles is one which provides these services.

146 Mary Shirley, "A behavior syndrome characterizing prematurely-born children," *Child Development* (Vol. 10, No. 2, June, 1939) pp. 118-119.

Chapter Four

Auditory

Do you hear noise in your head?
It pounds and screeches
Like a train rumbling through your ears
Do you hear noise in your head?

Do you see colours?
Swirling, twisting, stabbing at you
Like cuts on a movie screen hurling at you
Do you see colours?

Do you feel pain?
It invades every cell
Like an enemy unwanted
Do you feel pain?
Jeff Powell[147]

Touch may be the sense that has the biggest impact on the social development of the individual with autism, but hearing is the most difficult one to deal with. Auditory problems not only eliminate communication on a normal level, but also make sound almost impossible to escape. One can withdraw to avoid touch or smell. One can look down or close one's eyes to avoid using sight. One can refuse to taste by closing one's mouth, but there is no escape from sound. "It was the only thing that drove me crazy," claims Georgie Manly.[148]

For people, with a normal hearing range, super-hearing may seem desirable. Is it not the incredible ability we bestow on our superheroes such as the Six-Million Dollar Man or Superman? Have you ever taken the time to consider what super-hearing actually means? As you watch the television show where the superhero is able to turn up his hearing ability to the point that he is able to decipher a conversation in a house down the block, think about this. What happens to the sounds between the conversation and the superhero? Would not they also be amplified?

Watch a film taken in a classroom where children are involved in an activity between the camera and the viewer's point of focus. Not only are the sounds of the children present, the sounds are amplified and extremely irritating if you cannot see the cause.

Sit in a room and attempt to listen to a conversation in the next room with several people between you and the odour. Though they may appear to be sitting quietly, any noise they make becomes louder and a hindrance as you strain to hear the conversation. Even the turning of pages and the chewing of gum amplify to the point they obstruct your ability to hear.

These are only small examples of what the hearing experience is like to an individual with autism. Their acuity to sound is either on high or shut down. They can no more decrease the peripheral sounds in their daily life than we can ignore the pages being turned between us and the conversation next door. Everyday life for many individuals with autism is like living in the midst of a heavy metal rock concert. The normal everyday sounds we take for granted, such as the refrigerator motor, the furnace fan, or the clock ticking, are constantly annoying to those with hearing sensitivity. The sounds of our voices, of traffic, or the wind, are overwhelming: not because those who have autism have impaired hearing, but because they hear far too well.

In the past, focus on the auditory abilities of the autistic population has most often dealt with the theory that their hearing is disturbed or distorted. The observation that they respond to soft sounds while ignoring human voices or loud sounds is the basis of this consideration. If one takes the time to consider how well those who have autism really hear and what human voices sound like to them, one may get a more accurate picture of what is going on. One woman claims that as a young child "speech sounds just seemed to merge into one another without making any sense, a jumble of letters, hard to reproduce."[149] When we include in our understanding of autism the ability to block out the world, the lack of response to loud noises also begins to make far more sense.

In the film *A is for Autism*, the experience of hearing is described by a young man with autism as being like that of an untuned television[150]. Note that this description is one he has been told, not one that he developed himself. As I talked to this person and thought about his reactions and this description, I chose to try an experiment on myself. I turned the television on as loud as it would go. My teenage sons had connected extra speakers to the television at the time, so this was even louder than a normal television. The cartoon show *The Flintstones* was on. Fred and Barney were talking to each other and as I watched I caught the first half of a sentence. From then on the words started to pile up on one another and became jumbled together. I was unable to decipher anything they were saying. Within a few minutes the pain in my head was unbearable and I switched off the television. [151]

For the next two to three weeks, the pain returned whenever I heard a loud sudden noise, such as the banging of my kitchen cupboard doors. I believe that during this test, I experienced what the following young man describes.

> At the age of about two I could say a fair number of single words but hardly any full sentences. I was rarely able to hear sentences because my hearing distorted them. I was sometimes able to hear a word or two at the start and understand it and then the next lot of words sort of merged into one another and I could not make head nor tail of it. Darren White[152]

In the same way, Thomas McKean describes his experiences unloading a dishwasher after he thought auditory training had cured his hearing difficulties.

> I put the plates down on the shelf. The pain was almost unbearable. What happened? I thought I was over this! I walked over to the dishwasher, got some more plates and put them on the shelf, thinking it really didn't happen. It happened again. I stood quietly, looking at that monster that was the rest of the dishes. They looked back at me as if laughing at me in a merciless, malicious fashion. They looked back at me as if they knew they had won. I realized then that if I were the dishes, I would have done the same thing. I wondered why I had not thought to bring the ear protection I had always brought before. I finished the dishes. Very slowly.[153]

Last year I had the incredible experience of watching a child illustrate the reaction to distorted human speech in an unique manner. His mother was explaining to me how she felt he got nothing out of reading books. When he pretended to read them himself all he would do was make a line of sounds such as "da da da da." I asked her if she could try to show me what she was talking about. She sat down with her son and began to read a story to him as I watched.

After the mother had been reading awhile in her normal voice, she asked her son to read the page she had just read. He complied.

Child: "Put me da da da da da da da da da all."

At this point I asked the mother if she could read the next page in as soft a voice as possible. She read the next page, using a voice barely above a whisper: "Have no fear," said the Cat. "I will not let you fall."

When the child read this page after his mother, he repeated it word for word: "Have no fear," said the Cat. "I will not let you fall."

When one used a "normal" voice talking to this child, he could only pick out a few words at the beginning or end of a sentence. When one's voice was soft enough, he understood everything. The lack of response and the lack of learning this child revealed had nothing at all to do with cognitive effect, level of intelligence, or any disability. It was completely the result of the level of sound used in communication. This child had learned to communicate with only one or two words, not because he was incapable of learning anything else, but because that was how he heard communication. When he was speaking with people who were using their normal voices, he responded in the same way he heard them speak to him.

Little research has been carried out in the area of super-hearing, because most scientists do not believe it exists. Deafness has been recognized as a problem, and thus all children are tested to see if they are within the normal range of hearing. Few professionals take the time to go beyond the normal range to see what else may be out there. When one talks to a woman who as a small child could hear the bats scream (back in the forties before it was known that bats do make noises), it becomes obvious we are missing a lot of data. The puzzle of autism may begin to make more sense.

Individuals with Autism Say ...

> "She told me she was much more comfortable, that she no longer heard street noises three blocks away, or people flushing their toilets at the other end of the building, or the blood rushing in her veins......she hadn't been able to blow out the candles on her birthday cake because the sound of blowing had been so disturbing. "It sounded like monsters," she said, as had the puffing noise of the drain in the wall. People's breathing had upset her, especially when several adults were in the room.[154]
>
> The noises were bad too, not to be endured. Everyone talked in confusion, no beginning and no end was recognizable. It is no worse in a foreign country when one does not know the language." Dietmar Zoller[155]
>
> "Why do you think I have so much trouble paying attention in the classroom? I hear everything that goes on - every phone call that the principal makes in her office; every single time an eighteen-wheeler truck gears down on the highway three blocks away. I HEAR IT! I HEAR EVERYTHING! I hear people talking outside the school building, and I can understand their conversations. There are so many noises in my head that I can't concentrate on what Mrs. Weaver tries to say. I can't focus and pay attention to the teacher's spoken words - I'm too distracted. AND, why do you think I'm so tired all of the time? It takes so much energy to pay attention that I am worn out. I TRY SO HARD AND I JUST CAN'T DO IT!!!" Nicholas Bober[156]

Indications of Auditory Sensitivity

Watch for:

- The appearance of deafness. Those who have autism are not deaf; they have blocked out all sound.
- Grimaces when a sound occurs, or perhaps grimaces for no apparent reason.
- Echolalia, or the parroting back of what you have just said. This is an attempt by the person with autism to try to comprehend what you have said.
- Agitation or withdrawal from people who talk fast, talk constantly or talk loudly. Anxiety around people who have unusual vocal tones.
- Yelling on your part will lead to tantrums from them.
- Response to sounds you can't hear.

For example, while working at a group home out in the country, I dealt with a young man who would suddenly, for no apparent reason, become very obsessed with fire and begin lighting matches. It took the staff a long time to realize that every time this happened the fire alarm had gone off in the nearby town. We couldn't hear the siren; he could.

There are other sounds around us all the time, which we don't hear, but those who have autism respond to. One woman told me that when televisions are on, they produce a very high-pitched continuous hum. This is a sound most of us don't hear or even realize exists, so we don't take the time to consider its effect. As a child, this woman could walk past anyone's house and determine if the television was on. This sound may well be why some individuals with autism do not appear to enjoy watching television. It may also indicate why they will watch some sets, and not others.

Some children have trouble during the spring and summer months adjusting to the sounds of flying insects.[157]

Radios and televisions also cause problems as the commercials are produced at a higher decibel level than the regular programs.

Rooms with hard, shiny surfaces such as the tiles in bathrooms and kitchens may cause problems. Rooms that are sound absorbent (thick rugs, draperies, upholstered furniture) are much better.

Large, empty, echoing spaces can also be a problem. Examples are skating arenas, swimming pools, and shopping malls.

Mealtimes are often a problem with the clatter of cutlery and dishes, as well as the sounds people make when eating. Eating problems can occur due to sound. One lad told me he still doesn't eat celery at 17 because chewing it sounds like explosions going off in his head.

Some clothes can be noisy. Nylon pants and jackets are examples. They are going to be a problem whether they are worn by the person with autism, or by those who are working or playing with them. As one woman puts it, "If I take a walk in my new, quiet winter clothes next to someone wearing nylon clothing, I must walk 20 steps behind or ahead of the person."[158]

Sleeping problems can develop in noisy environments. Sources of the noise can be traffic, wind or motors that go off and on during the night, such those on furnaces and refrigerators.

Crowd conditions are extremely stressful. A lot of people talking at once is noted as unbearable by most individuals with autism. Applause can cause problems. Sudden bursts of laughter are overwhelming. The normal breathing pattern of people has also been mentioned as a problem. One high-functioning woman claims to be able to only deal with a maximum of four people at a time comfortably. The number is likely lower for those who are low functioning. The knowledge that one has absolutely no control over the noise level in a room and the fear that something is going to happen makes dealing with all social situations very difficult.

Individuals with hearing sensitivity may exhibit extreme reactions to loud sounds that may bother us, but that we have learned to deal with. For example:

> The smoke alarm, however, was a puzzle. Yes, it was loud, but he had heard it many times before, and at the age of five he would still have a reaction of blind hysteria. He would jump up, cover his ears, scream, run, spin around, run, spin around again, and run again. He was panic-stricken. He wanted to get away and didn't know how to get there.[159]

When your hearing is extremely acute, there is no way to "get used to" the pain these loud noises create. If you choose to expose someone with autism to these kinds of noises, be prepared to deal with effects, which could go on for weeks.

Loud, sudden blasts of noise, such as buzzers, horns, or balloons popping, are a problem. If a child is in an environment where this happens often, we may see no response at all to these noises. The child is likely to be constantly blocking out the sound by using repetitive stereotypic behaviours in order to protect himself.

Electric motors, especially those that have a high frequency sound, can send an individual with autism into a tailspin. For example: vacuum cleaners, blenders, electric saws, and fans in bathrooms. Heating and air conditioning systems are also often very noisy. The response is worse if the person has no idea that the noise is going to start.

The whistle of the wind, the patter of rain, even the wind moving through trees can be terrifying. Since these sounds are amplified, those who have autism often seem to be obsessed with the weather. This obsession is a means of protection from something they feel unable to control.

Traffic situations may be very dangerous as the person may well be blocking out sound and not hear what we think is very apparent.

Car travel may be a problem. The sound of the motor, the wind whistling past the windows, or the radio playing may all cause distress. These sounds, which can vary widely from one vehicle to the next, may well indicate why individuals with autism will ride in certain vehicles or with certain people, without a problem, and be totally disruptive in others. Travel problems can also be caused by tactile, visual or olfactory sensitivities.

The sound of running water is a huge problem. Fear in bathrooms is often connected directly to the sound of taps running. The sound of the toilet flushing and the echoes caused by tiled walls may also cause problems. The sound of waves on seashore may also be too much to bear.

Animals, especially dogs that bark a lot, may cause anxiety.

Haircuts can be very traumatic. The sound of the snipping scissors, and even more so, the sound of an electric clipper, is especially terrifying. Haircuts can also cause a problem with vision, touch and smell. Many people with autism report that having their hair cut is a very painful situation. They are unable to describe exactly what is causing the pain, but they know it hurts!

The runaway individual with autism is a cause for concern. These children often flee to avoid distressing noises. When looking for them, any further noise (calling) may make them retreat even further. We have to search in silence, which for us is very difficult.

Cleaning and washing ears is a problem. Ear infection is frequent.

People with autism often demonstrate perfect pitch. Some individuals have gone on as adults to find work as piano tuners. Many are gifted piano players and are able to transpose music from one key to another with no formal training. One child refused to play certain keys on his piano at home, as they were slightly out of tune, much to the consternation of his music teachers. As a preschooler, he would transpose his music lessons to another key in order to avoid hitting the keys that were not in tune. Instead of recognizing this behaviour as a talent, his teachers quit, because he was not following their instructions.

Reduced "P3Bs" amplitudes (neuophysiological activities in the brain triggered by internal mechanisms) for autistic subjects were measured in a study by Eric Courchesne, et al.[160] Similar findings in this area have been discovered in studies on normal adults with perfect pitch. The paper goes on to outline how the measurements gathered on autistic subjects reveal a disability in attention, which leads to the theory that autism is a devastating neurological disorder. However, these same measurements when found in "normal" adults reveal a gift! Where is the logic? When we discover the same data in two experiments, is it not probable that the results indicate a similar pattern? Perhaps the reduced P3Bs amplitude indicates that the individuals with autism in the study have perfect pitch. How can we help those who have autism when we cannot break through our own blindness and insist on finding a disability?

Method of Care

Never assume individuals with autism are deaf.

Never shout.

Never insist they listen to sounds they obviously don't like because you consider it is necessary for their development. It's like forcing a normal child to listen to someone running fingernails down a blackboard.

Speak as softly and as clearly as possible. Try whispering -- nonverbal children with autism have learned to speak through whispers.[161] However, for others, whispering is irritating because it accentuates the “s” sound.

I spent some time with a young lad who only spoke in one or two words, who never answered questions, and who used a lot of repetition. He was attending speech therapy at the local Health Unit where they believed that his problem was cognitive and that he was not able to understand what people were saying to him the first time they said it. Hours were spent holding his chin and repeating words, over and over and over in an effort to get him to learn.

When sitting at the dinner table with his family the conversation focused on the ability of people with autism to see in the dark. I turned to him and asked very softly (so softly that his mother who was sitting at the same table did not hear), "Do you like the dark, Robbie?" He replied "It is very beautiful, Gail." Does this boy have a cognitive problem? No! We are the ones who have the problem when we refuse to communicate with him in an appropriate manner.

Lowering one's voice often releases the person with autism from the need to use echolalia. Many of the autistic people I work with use echolalia with people who are talking in a normal level of voice, and reply directly to questions asked in a soft voice.

Use short, direct sentences. Do not chatter on and on. Do not repeat. Give the individual with autism time to decipher what you have said.

Respect the voice level of those who speak softly instead of insisting they "speak up". They are demonstrating the volume of speech, which is most comfortable for them. Lower your voice to match theirs.

Realize that when a person with autism is trying to communicate with you in sounds that are garbled, this is likely what you sound like to him. Through the understanding of body language and context, they have learned to decipher our messages. They respond to us like they hear. Our lack of comprehension becomes very puzzling and frustrating. If someone is "babbling" to you, it's a great sign, for they are trying to communicate. LOWER your voice when you talk to them so they can be free to learn to talk to us in a way we can understand. Tell them you can't understand because their speech is too loud. Never make fun of them or ignore them, or constantly tell them they are speaking incorrectly. If you do, they will give up trying to communicate.

In order to learn the social significance of language, and the proper use of the pronouns you, I and me, those who have autism need to hear the conversations of other people going on around them. Keep these conversations very soft, too.

Keep radios and televisions turned off as much as possible, as the difference in sound levels of commercials versus programming is too difficult. Use taped music instead so that the volume level can be kept constant. Allow the individual with autism to control the volume, if possible. If they turn it up very loud, be aware that they are likely using it as a means to cut off their hearing. Never, ever use radio or television as a constant background noise.

While in a doctor's office, a client sits quietly for a short time, and then begins to show signs of agitation such as squirming in his seat, flicking his fingers and tapping his feet. Instead of concentrating on the behaviour, I focus on the environment. A radio is playing. I ask to have it turned off. They comply. Another radio is playing. We locate it and have it turned off, too. Still another radio is playing. This is also turned off. The client then relaxes and sits quietly until the nurse calls his name.

Be aware of all noises around us. If possible, eliminate or try to muffle the household noises. Create an environment which is as absorbent to sound as possible. Close doors and windows; use heavy draperies, thick carpet and acoustic tiles in the ceilings.

Realize that these children also have to learn to cope with noise. If they are going to be part of regular society, exposure to regular noise levels is necessary. During this exposure, be aware they may need to react to sounds they cannot ignore. They will probably be less able to concentrate or learn new information in this situation.

A young man was being trained to work in a restaurant when he suddenly became very agitated and then quickly left. No one could understand just what had happened. A recording had been made of the training session. When the staff listened to the tape they could hear a women arguing loudly in the background. The trainer was able to block out these sounds as he concentrated on his task. The individual with autism could not.[162] This problem had nothing to do with ability; it was a problem with the sound levels. If the trainer had heard the argument at the same level as the person with autism, he would not be able to block it out either.

Cut down on mealtime noises with tablecloths, soft placemats, and "quiet" dishes (bang them against each other, and against cutlery to see which make the least noise).

Never use noise to "frighten" an individual with autism. Be aware that sudden, loud, unexpected noises are going to cause problems. On the other hand, regular loud noises may seem to go unnoticed due to sensory blocking. Be aware that a person with autism who is exposed to loud, sudden sounds must protect himself and cannot concentrate on anything else at the same time. Valuable school time and effort is wasted as the student prepares to block out the sound of the buzzers signalling the end of each class.

If one is building or renovating a home, consider installing a built-in vacuum so that the motor can be isolated away from the regular living area.

Those who have autism may be listening to sounds we cannot hear (fire sirens, helicopters, etc.) and may behave accordingly without us having any idea of what is going on. Our inability to hear the noise does not mean it is not occurring.

They may respond to certain places or events due to their history, such as once experiencing microphone feedback in a mall or a church. The noise level may not be painful in the present, but they will try to protect themselves anyway.

Keep them away from noisy places such as crowds, animals, and machinery as much as possible. When it is not possible, prepare them in advance for what is going to happen.

Prewarn them about noises that might bother them. Get them out of the room before we turn on the bath water, the blender, or an electric drill. Noises become such a common part of our environment that we may forget the stress they will cause an individual with autism. Try to be aware and prepare in advance. For example, the loud noise of a school buzzer may mean nothing more to us than freedom. Individuals with autism may have to prepare for the bell long in advance in order to protect themselves from pain. Is it necessary to ring so long and loud?

A child is in a kindergarten program. All is well as the class performs a song and dance for the rest of the school. At the end of the performance, the other students applaud enthusiastically. This child immediately responds with agitation, flapping his hands and looking for a way to run out.

By realizing that the applause will cause this type of reaction, we, as caregivers, can react with compassion and understanding instead of focusing on the undesirable behaviour. We may be ready to prepare the child for the noise in advance by covering his ears with our hands, or having him cover his own ears. After the noise has occurred, we may mention to him that it was stressful and that we are proud of the way he handled the situation. This gives the child the freedom to express his discomfort to us and the opportunity to learn ways to cope with the discomfort.

The human nervous system turns off when it cannot tolerate incoming noise. Individuals with autism may screech or scream for no apparent reason, using this as a method to block their sense of hearing. Sharing that their screeching hurts your ears seems to have a swift effect on eliminating this behaviour.

Soft music can be used to calm agitation. For some unknown reason, Beethoven seems to be particularly effective, especially his 9th Symphony, more commonly known as "*Ode to Joy*". However, as each person with autism is an individual, they should be free to choose their own favourites. For example, Sara Miller finds classical music very soothing and relaxing, but cannot tolerate the sound of brass instruments, even when they are in the classics.[163] Individuals with autism may use music to block out the world, so watch that it is not overdone.

If a person with autism has been exposed to an especially loud and painful noisy situation, the effects may go on for two or three weeks. They will be sensitive to noises that usually do not seem to bother them. They may also be more tuned out during this period.

Time-outs in a quiet space may be effective for calming agitation caused by noise. Earplugs might be useful in situations such as skating arenas or malls. If there is a tactile sensitivity, the individual with autism may not be able to cope with earplugs. Earmuffs might also be useful, but again may cause tactile problems.

There are new devices called noise suppressors on the market. These devices block out background noise so that one is able to concentrate more fully. The sound of a person speaking directly to you is not blocked out, but is muted to the point that the sound of the voice is comfortable. One product like this, that I have tried and found comfortable and effective, is the Noisebuster. It is available through Noise Cancellation Technologies, Inc., One Dock Street, Suite 300, Stamford, CT, 06902. Telephone (800) 278-3526 or (203) 961-0500. The price is about $79.00 US. It was originally recommended to me by a person with autism. Others have tried it and found it to their liking.

Time spent out in nature, away from the noises of city life, is beneficial.

Teach songs very softly on an individual basis, in order that the student might later sing along with a group. Be prepared to have a negative reaction to your singing, if you are unable to stay on key. Having perfect pitch means that singing or playing off key is extremely irritating to individuals with autism.

Never forget that all lessons learned will be affected by the ability to hear well. For example: one mother was trying to teach her child a common lesson we all learn - to stop, look and listen before crossing the street. She practiced it time and again with her son before they went out to attempt it in traffic and she felt that he understood clearly. However, when they came to the edge of the street and stopped, looked (nothing coming) and listened, he refused to cross the street. This mother had the advantage of having a high-functioning adult with autism to consult with and went to her with the problem. Why did her son refuse to cross the street? The woman answered, "If you wait long enough, the car will come." His hypersensitive hearing meant that he could hear cars approaching long before they were in sight. The “listen” part of the lesson became a problem for the boy, because he could hear too well.[164]

Group story reading is rather a waste of time if you want the individual with autism to understand the story, as it will be too loud to decipher. Read very softly in an individual situation. On the other hand, group stories are beneficial for teaching social interaction.

Try to have quiet interaction between the child with autism and other children, during quiet periods as well as during free time at school. They may be trying to interact with other children, but cannot understand them when they talk in their normal voices. Reinforce talking softly, perhaps by making a game of it. Whispering is a good idea between children when you are working with them. Information must be given in a very soft voice if the individual with autism is going to understand it.

When you don't understand what is happening with the individual with autism, admit it to them. Remember to make all statements and ask all questions in a very soft voice.

Do not use repetition. Lower your voice and try new phrases and words. Never parrot what they say to us. Develop new phrases to make the message clearer. This is especially important with children who have been exposed to therapy where repetition has played a major role.

Ignore any loud talk after telling them to use a quiet voice. Respond when they speak quietly. Keep voices quiet so they can learn to be quiet too. Their loudness may be an attempt to try to respond as they hear us speak.

Always share our feelings with them so they can learn to share theirs with us.

Allow a person with autism to have the right to his or her own feelings. If they say they are able to hear something long before we do, such as a train approaching, respect this ability. Don't put them down by refusing to believe them, or perhaps telling them that they cannot "hear" the sound but must be sensing it.[165] Those who have autism are not aliens -- they are human beings just like you and me. Would we do this to a teenager if he claimed to hear something before his grandfather did? Of course not. Use the same respect with people with autism you show anyone else. The ability to hear well may also be used as a special gift. Perhaps you can give them the job of "hearing" Dad drive down the street first.

Never forget that all behaviour is a method of communication of some sort. Expect individuals with autism to communicate with us in whatever way they can. Do not just do things for them. Let them make choices and decisions. Be patient and wait until they do so.

Watch the children closely to see if they have developed their own methods of communication which we may not have been party to. While playing with his cousin in his room, a boy with autism and a "normal" girl were observed whispering to each other. This boy really enjoyed having the little girl visit. It was obvious that the two of them had worked out their own solution to communication, one that included him fully.

People who suffer from hyperacusis (see Chapter 1 for more information on this condition) have developed their own network to develop solutions to their hypersensitivity to noise. If you are working with, or the parent of, someone who has problems with sound, it might be wise to join this network. Regular newsletters are published which offer all sorts of helpful hints, from the quietest kinds of appliances, computers, and vehicles available, to hints on how to deal with noise from the environment, to what kind of devices, such as ear plugs and noise suppressors, are most effective. You can reach the Hyperacusis Network at 444 Edgewood Drive, Green Bay, WI 54302.

Conclusion

One of the most difficult areas in auditory care is changing the behaviours of the caregivers. Even when parents and professionals recognize super sensitivity, others, who provide the daily care for the individual, can impede any progress. A mother called me to share her experiences and those of her daughter. The daughter's sensitivity to sound had been recognized by family members. The mother was fortunate enough to find an audiologist who was willing to listen to her concerns and test her daughter above the normal range of hearing. As a professional, he recommended that this young girl wear earplugs at all times to protect her from the noise in the environment. Her teachers refused to allow her to use the earplugs in the classroom. Even with letters from both the parents and the doctor, the teachers continued in their own way. They chose to believe that the girl was using her hearing difficulties as an excuse to get out of work, rather than respect the painful reality she was experiencing.

Hearing has been described by individuals with autism as the cause of most problems in their lives. Controlling the noise levels in their environments has proved to be impossible. They are constantly assaulted by too much sound. Simple things to us, like breathing, the wind, and the sound of running water may terrify them. Sound not only causes pain, but it also intensifies the level of anxiety, as those who have autism worry about where the noise is coming from and what is going to happen next. This anxiety often develops into what we define as a fixation, such as with weather conditions.

Problems with hearing directly lead to problems with communication. Lack of effective communication is the most frustrating factor in an autistic experience. Lack of an appropriate method of communication is a big part of the "abnormal" behaviour patterns of the autistic population. Studies have indicated that if certain abilities such as language have not been acquired by a critical age (seven), the more difficult it will be for them to be learned.[166] However, one must realize that these studies focus on individuals who had absolutely no access to language until they were older than seven, and on their ability to learn a foreign language. A child with autism has been exposed to language from birth, but often does not react like we want because the language he hears is not directed at him, it comes from the distance. Because they have receptive language abilities, they may often begin to speak later than seven.

Hearing is also extremely important for learning. Most of the information we absorb comes to us through the use of our ears. How can anyone be expected to learn if the information they receive is coming in too loudly to decipher?

It is imperative we speak softly to people with autism if we want them to understand everything we are saying. It is also imperative to speak softly if we want those who have autism to learn the information we are providing. If we insist on using our normal voice, we are wasting our time and theirs. If we shout, we are putting them through torture, and they should have the right to let us know it, regardless of which communication method they choose to use. This is likely the most important message you will get from reading this book.

I do realize there are many people, especially teachers and speech therapists, who will read this advice and reject it outright. Since it was never taught to them in college, they may think it cannot be that important. But believe me, it is.

I also realize that the dramatic story recorded earlier of the young lad who answered my question so easily, is not going to happen to each and every child with autism. However, speaking softly to them does work, sometimes immediately, with others over longer periods of time. There are many reports of children obeying a command for the first time in their lives when their parents tried speaking softly to them. For other children, there is no other response than a look on their face, which indicates that a window of understanding has been opened.

Some children begin to babble more and more, once people around them start speaking in a soft voice. Gradually words emerge from the babbling and these children embark on the road to verbal communication. Others use echolalia when spoken to in a normal or loud tone of voice, but respond to the communication when a soft tone is used. Other parents do not report anything so dramatic, but note that their child has become less and less frustrated with life as people speak softly to him.

Speaking softly is an easy gift we can choose to give people with autism. It doesn't cost anything. It takes even less energy than speaking in a loud or normal voice. It will never hurt the child in any way. And yet, there are many who resist. It is time for you to question just why you resist at such a simple measure. Yes, we may have to break a lifelong habit of speaking louder when we think someone does not understand us. Is that so difficult?

One of the interesting aspects of the integration of these children into the regular school system is the teacher's aide sitting close by the student with autism relaying the information from the classroom teacher. The teacher's aide speaks very softly, not for the benefit of the student, but to not bother the rest of the classroom. Inadvertently, this aide is providing her student with a message that can be clearly deciphered by the student affected with autism.

In order to give people with autism the chance to be as normal as possible, please speak softly. If we make this choice, we can share with them the gift of verbal communication.

147 Jeffery Powell, Jr., Baldwinsville, New York. Used with permission.

148 Annabel Stehli, *The Sound of a Miracle* (New York: Doubleday, 1991) p. 188.

149 Therese Jolliffe, Richard Lansdown and Clive Robinson, "Autism: a personal account," *Communication* (Vol. 26, no.3, 1992) p. 13.

150 Dick Arnall (producer) and Tim Webb (director), *A is for Autism* (London: Finetake Production for Channel 4, 1992). For a unique visual illustration of this experience on hearing and speech see this film. Available for rent from Film Makers Library, Room 901, 124 East 40th Street, New York, NY 10016, Phone: 212-808-4980, Fax: 212-808-4983.

151 Under no condition would I advise anyone to try this experiment on themselves.

152 B.B. While and M.S. Whilte, "Autism from the inside," *Medical Hypothesis* (Vo. 24, 1987) p. 224.

153 Thomas McKean, "An insider look at auditory training," *The Advocate* (Vol. 25, no.1, 1993) p. 14.

154 Annabel Stehli, p. 171.

155 Dietmar Zoller, *Wenn ich mit euch redden konnte...* (Bern, Germany: Scherz Verlag, 1989) Introduction translated by Annie Humphreys of the Autism Research Unit, Sunderland Polytechnic, Sunderland, Great Britain.

156 Sally Bober, "Nicholas", *Dancing in the Rain*, edited by Annabel Stehli (Westport, CT: The Georgiana Organization, Inc., 1995) pp.114-115.

157 Jean Jasinski, "Jason", *Dancing in the Rain*, edited by Annabel Stehli (Westport, CT: The Georgiana Organization, Inc., 1995) p. 4.

158 Connie Schwarting, "Loud Clothing", *Hyperacusis Network* (March, 1996), p.3.

159 Kendra Marasco, "Joey", *Dancing in the Rain*, edited by Annabel Stehli (Westport, CT: The Georgiana Organization, Inc., 1995) p. 54.

160 Eric Courchesne, Alan Lincoln, Rachel Young-Courchesne, Roberta Elmasian, and Christian Grillon, "Pathophysiologic findings in nonretarded autism and receptive developmental language disorder," *Journal of Autism and Developmental Disorders* (Vol. 19, no. 1, 1989) p. 12.

161 Jack Copeland, *For the Love of Ann Based on the Diary of Jack Hodges* (London, Severn House Publishers, 1976).

162 Deborah Pearce, "Shifting world of autism tricks the senses," *Times-Colonist* (Victoria, B.C.: 1991, September 20) p. C3.

163 Sara Miller, "Does the Princess have PDD? Family Gatherings," *Autism Society of Northeastern Wisconsin Newsletter* (November, 1993).

164 Carol Meredith, Denver, CO, Personal communication.

165 Laura Cesaroni and Malcolm Garger, "Exploring the experience of autism through firsthand accounts, " *Journal of Autism and Developmental Disorders* (Vol. 21, no.3, 1991) p. 306.

166 E. Mavis Hetherinton and Ross Parke, *Child Psychology: A Contemporary Viewpoint* (New York: McGraw-Hill Book Company, 1989) p. 288.

Chapter Five

Visual

A father shows his son a flock of geese flying by. To his dismay, the boy refuses to look in the direction of the geese, but he does point at them.

A mother spends all her free time with her son who has autism, trying to make eye contact. This mother firmly believes that once her child can look deeply into her eyes for a length of time, they will be able to make progress in the areas of social awareness, communication and emotional development.

On a bright sunny day a child runs screaming from the side of a lake. He approaches his therapist, demanding she repeat addresses he is obsessed with, as he rubs his face. In a desire to help, but totally puzzled, she yells at him that she cannot help if he does not tell her what is wrong. Startled, he replies that she must get the thing that hurts out of his eye. For the first time in their association, the therapist realizes that this lad feels visual pain.[167]

The visual experience of individuals with autism and those who care for them can be described in many different ways. The father wants to share his joy in nature with his son and is terribly frustrated that the son refuses to look. The mother is certain that the eyes must be used as the starting point to build a relationship. The therapist is so caught up with the psychoanalysis of the boy's bizarre behaviours and what she feels is the obsessive repetition of words that she misses the messages he is sharing. All three of these caregivers are lost in their own misconceptions. Perhaps in each case the situation has a visual meaning being missed by all of them.

Descriptions of the visual problems of individuals with autism, by "normal" people and then by people with autism themselves, are the farthest removed in content and recognition of the problem. We "normal" people see the biggest obstacle in vision as the lack of eye contact[168] and the behaviour of "looking through" people.[169] Individuals with autism, on the other hand, describe the joy they get looking at things that we do not even consider interesting. Grains of sand, the grooves in one's fingerprint, and colours in a puddle may be fascinating to them.[170] These descriptions, of course, come from those who are high-functioning enough to be able to describe their visual experiences accurately. Others are believed to be legally blind and function as such. Who knows what they see when they look at the world?

Visual problems described by individuals with autism include the blurring of colours, the apparent change in size of objects, and the uncomfortable feeling they have when looking at certain things. Other experiences are more like horror shows. Donna Williams vividly describes the feeling of visual over stimulation in the book *Somebody Somewhere.*

> Dr. Marek's kitchen was a nightmare. The kitchen had fluorescent lights and yellow walls, one of the worst combinations ever. Even from the doorway I could see light bouncing off everything.
>
> In my tense state everything climbed to hyper, vision included. There were no whole objects in that room, just shiny edges and things that jumped off the yellow walls like sunshine on water. Dr. Marek wanted me to go in there and be blind. Forget it!
>
> I stood in the doorway looking at the light, my eyes jumping from half object to half object trying to take things in. Maybe I could relax a bit and

> pay attention to this person I was supposed to meet. She was Mrs. Marek, a face upon which light danced maniacally, turning her into more of a cartoon than a human being. Welcome to *Toon Town*, Roger Rabbit. I'd like you to enter this torture chamber I call my kitchen and meet my wife, who is a 3-D cartoon. She just wants you to look at her in pieces, say hi whether you mean it or not, and treat her like a human being.[171]

As one considers the visual experience of the person with autism, one must have some understanding of how the eye works. The eye has two kinds of visual receptors, rods and cones.[172] The cones function under daylight conditions and are non-functional at night. The rods, on the other hand are responsible for night vision. The cones are located in the centre of the visual field, the fovea. Their number gradually decreases as one moves to the periphery or edge of the retina. There are no rods in the fovea of the eye. Their number increases as one moves to the outer edge of the retina.

As with their other senses, the acuity of vision of the individual with autism is heightened. More stimulation occurs when a person with autism looks at something; pain is the result if the stimulation is too intense. Look directly into the bright lights of oncoming traffic or try to pick out the features of a person standing in front of a sunlit window and experience this discomfort. To lessen the pain, people with autism learn to use their peripheral vision (a low amount of cones, plus rods) and as a result, they appear to us to be looking off to one side when they are actually looking at something or someone.

As caregivers for individuals with autism, the use of peripheral vision is a very important factor to consider. Insistence that those who have autism look directly at an object or an activity may mean we are insisting that they do not see. Waiting until they look directly at the task may well mean that time is wasted while they, with their peripheral vision, are already doing what we ask. I realize it is hard to try and comprehend just what they are seeing and how they are doing it. But I definitely feel it is more useful to err on the side of false expectation than to waste their childhood waiting for a child to look in the direction we want.

Sensory integration specialists spend a lot of time and effort training individuals with autism to use their central vision. People who have gone through this training may adapt to doing tasks in front of them, but they also claim they no longer see clearly. Their vision is blurred and often cuts out altogether. In order to appear normal, those who have autism have been robbed of their sight. Is that what we really want for them?

There are also problems for individuals with autism when they use their peripheral vision to see. The centre of the scene is blurred while the edges are in focus. Drawings by children with autism often illustrate this reaction. The animated film *A is for Autism*[173] has several examples of this effect. Those who have autism also find it difficult to locate objects they want to see, as well as determining and remembering the distinct features of faces.

Eye contact is so often stressed as a necessity to reaching anyone socially. With the individual with autism, we again may be doing more harm than good when we insist on eye contact. The heightened arousal that people with autism are unable to cope with, and, therefore must block out, is probably not worth our satisfaction of gaining contact. The increased level of acuity means that those who have autism are seeing more in our eyes than we see when we look into theirs. Georgie Manly is bothered by the movement and colours of our eyes when she looks into them.[174] Why do we need to insist on this contact if it is causing them stress? Give them time to choose to make it themselves, and be prepared for only short periods of eye contact. If this is all they can endure, the empathy we share with them is worth far more than any direct eye contact.

Facilitated Communication is a method of communication being used with individuals with autism, in which typewriters, computers or other message boards allow the person to spell out a message.[175] To many people, this method of communication is a miracle. To others, it is meaningless manipulation of the person with autism by the facilitator. One of the main arguments quoted is that the individual with autism may not look at the keyboard when putting in the messages.[176] We must recognize that this behaviour ties directly to the use of peripheral vision. As we look at the angle of sight used by those who have autism, it may be very difficult to understand how they are able to see the keyboard. Again we must make the effort to respect their abilities, rather than insisting on our own definition of the situation.

Another feature of our visual system is the ability to create pictures in our own mind of what we are about to see. When we enter a room that we have visited in the past, our visual picture comes into play. If the room has changed dramatically, the visual picture is out of sync with our visual reality. People with autism, who may have stronger feelings than we do, and who are not prepared for the change that will meet their eyes, will react far more dramatically than we do. The contrast between the visual picture and the visual reality is so great that their system will overload. Fear and the need for protection will dominate their behaviour.[177]

It is important to prepare individuals with autism for any change of this nature. If that is impossible, the ability to recognize that the fear is caused by the visual contrasts gives us the chance to empathize with the person. It is best to remove them from the scene for a period of time to allow them to calm down, and then slowly reintroduce them to the situation so they have the time to adjust their visual picture.

Individuals with Autism Say ...

> Each particle of sand intrigued me as though I were a scientist looking through a microscope. Other times I scrutinized each line in my finger, following one as if it were a road on a map. Temple Grandin[178]

> I also remember one Christmas when I got a new bike for a present. It was yellow. I would not look at it. Extra red was added to the colour making it look orange and it blurred upwards making it look like it was on fire. My favourite colours were those I could see more clearly than others. I also couldn't see blue clearly, it looked too light and it looked like ice (imagine the sea on a sunny day, it would look frozen over, in spite of the sun). The bike was painted purple, which I liked better because I could see it more clearly. Darren White[179]

> It is my wish to campaign for understanding for autistics. No one knows what it means to be disturbed in perception. I remember that before, all people had a crooked nose and looked bad, even my mother whom I loved so much later. People were monsters, forms made out of fat without contours. Dietmar Zoller[180]

> The eye examination is to find out if i see too much my eyes often hurt and i see everything it is very hard to bear inside me i can simply switch it off and within seconds all i see is a high wall of dots. Birger Sellin[181]

Indications of Visual Sensitivity

Watch for:

- Apparent blindness.
- Closed eyes, or eyes rolled up so only the whites show.
- Looking past people or seemingly through people.
- Pointing directly at something while looking off in another direction.
- Looking off to one side rather than straight ahead while walking, riding a tricycle, watching television, or doing a task.
- Fear of bright shiny objects, of mirrors and often certain colours, or of different colour combinations.
- Squinting.
- Attempts to mould the faces of caregivers.
- Constantly having to touch the environment, such as running one's hands along the walls as one walks down a hall.
- Agitation when exposed to bright lights, bright sunlight, brightly lit rooms. The sun shining on large surfaces of water or on new snow is especially painful.
- Agitation or refusal to comply when exposed to certain colours. The problem colour will vary from one individual to another. Red and yellow are often noted to cause the most problems.
- Long periods of time spent staring directly into a bright light.
- Finger fiddling in front of the eyes, spinning objects, fascination with fans or other moving objects.
- Fascination with spinning objects, such as tops, lids, the wheels of toy cars, or records and cassette tapes.
- Fascination with fans or other moving objects.
- Fear of heights, stairs, dark tunnels, and movement.
- Rubbing, touching or hitting the eyes. Rubbing the face.
- Sleeping problems.
- Agitation in environments that are loaded with visual stimuli, especially moving stimuli.
- Agitation in rooms in which fluorescent lighting is used.
- Poor depth perception problems occur when getting on elevators, walking down stairs, catching balls, bumping into things, or walking over objects without apparently seeing them.

Method of Care

Never assume that the individual with autism is blind. Also, never assume that the individual with autism is not looking at you, the task, or where he is pointing even though it appears to you that he is not. Respect his use of peripheral vision.

Never force an individual with autism to look directly at a task or at what you are teaching. You may be making them miss out on the information you are trying to provide. Do not wait to teach until you have them looking directly at what you are teaching. You are only wasting time.

Keep the environment as neutral and empty as possible in order to eliminate visual over stimulation.

Never use bright lights or bright, shiny objects. If possible, eliminate all fluorescent lights. These lights flicker constantly, driving people with acute vision to distraction.

Consider the colours, or the combination of colours of objects, clothing or a room, especially if the child appears fearful. For example red and yellow may look like flames. Different colours seem to cause trouble for different individuals. There seems to be a connection with true colours versus mixtures or blended colours, much like the problem with perfect pitch in the auditory area, but this has never been measured. One woman feels nauseous every time she looks at the colours red and green next to each other. One young man claims that bright yellow is hard for him to deal with.[182] Another claims to have problems with pale blue as it reminds him of the sun shining on water.[183]

Watch which clothes you expect them to wear and also what you are wearing. Neutral colours (earth tones) seem to be the best. A mother went shopping with her daughter and noticed an increased level of agitation as the day progressed. The daughter kept saying the word "red" and the mother responded by trying to find red outfits for the daughter to try on. This just led to increased agitation and the mother realized that it was best to take her daughter home. In this safe environment, she was able to explain that her mother's red silk blouse was driving her crazy. If you work with individuals with autism, when choosing a wardrobe, it seems best to choose neutral colours such as earth tones until you know what effect colour has on the individual you are working with.

Colours in the environment also make a difference. A teacher papered sections of the walls in her classroom over the weekend in a bright red, blue and yellow in an attempt to make the room more stimulating. Daily schedules were posted on a yellow section of the wall. One child absolutely refused to go near the schedule, covering his eyes with his hands and turning away. Once the yellow paper was removed, he no longer showed this reaction. Later it was noted that many of the tasks he had trouble with, and often refused to do, had bright yellow components.

Staring directly into bright light allows the child to cut off stimulation. Therefore do not allow it; redirect them to another activity. Sunglasses are a necessity on bright days, especially near surfaces of water or on bright, sunny, winter days. Tactile problems may well come into effect here, so be aware that they may be the reason the individual with autism is rejecting the sunglasses. For people with severe vision problems, wearing sunglasses at all times may help.

When teaching, never hold the lessons near your face. The individual with autism has trouble concentrating on the two stimuli simultaneously.[184]

While working on tasks, have a blank neutral wall in front of the person with autism, not a whole room of stimulation.[185]

It is better to use books and illustrations with small writing and pictures, than books that have been enlarged. The smaller the better.

Problems with reading may have to do with the paper one is dealing with. A young lad claimed "I can't read this cheap book - I need to get the hardbound copy." When asked why he said that, he explained he could see the words from the other side of the page coming through the page he was trying to read.[186]

Before going to bed have the child spend some time in a very dimly lit environment. This allows the production of serotonin to slow down. While sleeping, keep the room pitch dark.

Do not worry about the child being in the dark. They can see much better than we can with very little light. One child reads with only the light coming in the crack under her bedroom door at night. Another child was able to pick up a handful of pills his mother had dropped on the floor before she was able to switch on the lights. It was too dark for the mother to see anything. Let them take pride in this ability.

Do not insist on eye contact. Individuals with autism say that the colours in our eyes move and flicker, making them feel very uncomfortable. Forcing them to have eye contact with us is regarded as an intrusion into their core being. When they are ready for eye contact, they will give it to you.

When first coming in contact with an autistic child, try using peripheral vision in order to allow the child to make the first contact and give them the feeling that you do understand.[187]

While talking to individuals with autism, do not look directly at them but at something else; out the window, or perhaps at a picture on the wall, in order that they may concentrate on your message.[188]

Haircuts may be a problem due to the use of bright shiny scissors, bright lights, and many mirrors. Agitation during haircuts may also stem from odour (yours), sound, and touch. For sight, try dull-finished or painted scissors and eliminate the mirrors.

Obsessive interest in an object we see as boring may be due to features that we are unable to see. Talk about it. One may be very surprised at the result.

Be aware that using a two-way window-mirror to observe these individuals may not be beneficial. They may be watching us as we watch them.

Allow people with autism extra time to explore new surroundings, preferably when there are few other people present, in order for them to develop a visual map of the area.

The use of Irlen lenses may prove helpful to those who are having problems with their vision. The Irlen method uses colour to alleviate perceptual distortions.[189] Each individual is measured to find the colour which is best suited to his own eyes. The tints in different glasses may vary from rosy pink to brown to blue.

I personally support the use of Irlen lenses for many reasons. They are an improvement on my suggestion to use sunglasses and cut down on the amount of light that is entering the eyes. They do not claim to be a "cure" for autism, but are used as another way for people with sensory sensitivities to cope with the environments they live in. And most of all, they are recommended by many people with autism who have chosen to try them, including Thomas McKean, Sharisa Joy Kochmeister, Donna Williams and Richard Attfield.

> I looked in quick glances, understood by piecing fragments. I saw cracked children, cracked steps, print and writing. Since having tinted lenses I have the sight and hearing I very much wanted. Richard Attfield.[190]

> For me, the effects of Irlen Lenses were shattering. My two dimensional world, without depth perception, suddenly looked three dimensional. It didn't look like a picture anymore, it looked like a place. My husband wasn't a collection of disconnected floating facial features; he was a whole connected face, taken in not bit by bit, but as a whole. Things weren't all there by coincidence anymore. Understanding wasn't a struggle.

> The result for me is that the processing involved for depth perception and coherence of visual information improved dramatically, among other things. I now am rarely meaning-blind and don't have to touch everything to know where I am in space. I feel more secure in my less fragmented environment and around what are now less fragmented people. I have more time to grasp my thoughts and feelings and my other senses, and since I no longer have to compensate for visual overload, I can also keep up better with processing sound, touch, or body connectedness. Donna Williams[191]

There are many Irlen Clinics operating throughout the world. A list of their locations, as well as more information on this method, can be obtained from Helen Irlen, 5380 Village Road, Long Beach, CA 90808. The telephone number is (562) 496-2550.

Conclusion

Visual sensitivity is very important to the individual in any area of learning. If they cannot see what we are trying to teach them, they cannot learn as well. If they are using peripheral vision and we are insisting they use direct gaze, we may be depriving them of the chance to learn what we are trying to teach. If the room is too bright, they may not see anything at all. If they are overwhelmed by visual stimulation, they may need to escape into repetitious behaviour to protect themselves. As caring, aware teachers, we can turn their world around.

Snow blindness is a unique condition which results when a person spends too much time out in the bright sunlight in a snow covered setting. The reflection of the sun on the white snow temporarily damages the eyes. This damage may last up to one week. A snow-blind person may have trouble distinguishing colours or may see everything as the colour red. In most cases, resting the eyes and staying indoors is all that is required to solve the problem.[192] A similar condition, called welder's blindness, occurs when one looks at a welder's arc without proper protection.

Individuals with autism who are declared legally blind may well be suffering from a form of snow blindness (without the snow).[193] The intensity of the normal light in our environment may be producing the same reaction for those who have autism as the sun reflecting on the snow does on those who experience actual snow blindness. There is a definite need for research in this area.

Serotonin is a biochemical in the brain which is produced in the pineal gland. In mammals, the amount of serotonin produced by this gland is directly determined by the amount of light taken in by the eyes.[194] Autistic subjects have been measured and found to have high levels of serotonin as compared to normal subjects.[195] These high levels may well suggest that the eyes of individuals with autism process more light. During the day serotonin is produced by the pineal gland. During the night, or while we are sleeping, the serotonin is changed to melatonin, a hormone which makes people drowsy.[196]

Since some individuals with autism have a high level of serotonin in their systems combined with an ability to process even low levels of light, it is possible that sleep patterns will be affected. In order to produce the melatonin needed to feel drowsy, autistic people need access to very dim areas before they are sent to bed. They also should sleep in total darkness in order that serotonin production does not start up again. Administration of a synthetic melatonin has proved to help some people with autism sleep better.[197]

167 Mira Rothenberg, *Children with Emerald Eyes* (New York: E.P.Dutton, 1987) p. 248.

168 Patricia Mirenda, Anne Donnellan and David Yoder, "Gaze behavior: A new look at an old problem," *Journal of Autism and Developmental Disorders* (Vol. 13, no. 4, 1983) p. 397.

169 Ruth Sullivan, *Definition of Autism* (Huntington, West Virginia: Autism Services Center, 1988) p. 1.

170 Temple Grandin & Margaret Scariano, *Emergence: Labeled Autistic* (Novato, California, Arena Press, 1986) p. 22.

171 Donna Williams, *Somebody Somewhere* (Toronto, Ontario: Doubleday Canada Limited, 1994) p. 94-95.

172 Donald McBurney & Virginia Collings, *Introduction to Sensation/ Perception* Second Edition (Englewood Cliffs, N.J.: Prentice-Hall Inc. 1984) pp. 55-60.

173 Dick Arnall (producer) and Tim Webb (director), *A is for Autism* (London: A Finetake Production for Channel 4, 1992).

174 Annabel Stehli, The Sound of a Miracle (New York: Doubleday, 1991) p. 188.

175 Douglas Biklen, "Communication Unbound: Autism and Praxis," *Harvard Educational Review* (Vol. 60, no. 3, 1990) pp. 291-314.

176 Jon Palfreman, Producer and Director, "Prisoners of Silence," *Frontline* (Boston, WGBH Educational Foundation, October 1, 1993).

177 Sara Miller, Does the Princess have PDD? "Visual Sensitivity" (unpublished manuscript).

178 Temple Grandin and Margaret Scariano, p. 22.

179 Darren White, More Autobiography (unpublished manuscript).

180 Dietmar Zoller, *Wenn ich mit euch redden konnte...* (Bern: Germany, Scherz Verlag, 1989). Introduction translated by Annie Humphreys of the Autism Research Unit, Sunderland Polytechnic, Sunderland, Great Britain.

181 Birger Sellin, *I don't want to be inside me anymore* (New York: Basic Books, 1995) p. 138.

182 Thomas McKean, "An alternate look at autistic perceptions," in *Proceedings from Autism: A World of Options Conference* (Toronto: Autism Society of America and Autism Society Canada, July, 1993) p. 30.

183 Darren White, More Autobiography (unpublished manuscript).

184 Temple Grandin, "Defensiveness-research findings, sensory problems and sensory stimulation," (Cassette recording) Autism Society of America Conference (Los Angeles, California: July, 1990). Tape available from the Educational Audio Recording Service, P.O. Box 720135, Houston, Texas 77272.

185 Amy Lettick, "On structuring a lesson," *Journal of Learning Disabilities* (Vol. 6, no. 1, 1973) p. 12.

186 Sally Bober, "Nicholas", *Dancing in the Rain*, edited by Annabel Stehli (Westport, CT: The Georgiana Organization, Inc.), 1995) p. 118.

187 Patricia St. John, *The Secret Language of Dolphins* (New York, Summit Books, 1991) p. 184.

188 Donna Williams, *Nobody Nowhere* (Toronto, Doubleday, Canada Limited, 1992) p. 216.

189 Helen Irlen, "I can't stand the bright lights: breaking free from perceptual-sensory distortion" *A New Dawn of Awakening*, Autism Society of America Conference proceedings (Arlington, TX: Future Horizons, Inc., 1994) pp. 259-261. See also: Helen Irlen's book *Reading by the Colors*, Avery Press.

190 Helen Irlen, P. 260.

191 Donna Williams, "The lived experience of Irlen filters", *Advocate* (newsletter) Autism Society of America, Inc. (Nov-Dec, 1995) p. 7.

192 Ron Klein, "Snow blindness," *The World Book Encyclopedia* Volume 17 (Toronto: World Book Inc. 1991) p. 540.

193 Thanks to Randy Gillingham for suggesting this connection.

194 Bruce Fellman, "A clockwork gland," *Science 85* (Vol.6, no. 4, 1985) p. 79.

195 E. Ritvo and B.J. Freeman, "A medical model of autism: etiology, pathology and treatment," *Pediatric Annals* (Vol. 13, no. 4, 1984) p. 300.

196 Bruce Fellman, p. 80.

197 Personal communication with Dr. Keith Golden, Glenrose Hospital, Edmonton, Alberta Canada.

Chapter Six

Olfactory

Smell is the sense which is most likely to be ignored by people who are working with individuals with autism, and yet is one which is very important, because it can cause a great deal of stress. When we smell, the molecules of odour are absorbed directly through the nasal cavity to the receptor cells of the olfactory nerves.[198] These fifty million neurons, otherwise known as cilia, are replaced every thirty days so they are strong and effective throughout our lives. They are the most exposed of our neurons, sticking out and waving in the air currents of our breath. Messages are sent straight to the limbic system of the brain, the centre of all feeling. With every breath of air we flood this sensory system with odour. If we stop breathing, we die.

For various reasons, there is less known about the sense of smell than any of the other senses.[199] The location and size of the receptors, the quality of the stimuli and the ability to send a certain quantity in order to measure the response are only some of the difficulties encountered by scientists.

For a person who has a stronger reaction to odour, any environment can be overwhelming. Many of our perfumes are fabulous only when diluted. They can be repulsive if too strong or if combined with other odours. Smell triggers memories faster and more effectively than any other sense.[200] Agitation, due to painful memories, may often occur even if the odours are pleasant at that moment.

Smell is also one of the first senses we rely on during our life. Studies with newborn infants have found that they show preference for certain odours and find others nauseating. They will turn away from unpleasant odours shortly after birth and can recognize their mothers by smell.[201] This may well account for the problem that some of these supersensitive babies have during breast feeding. A strong sense of smell, combined with tactile defensiveness, can easily explain the need to withdraw.

These problems of infancy can last throughout a lifetime. I spoke with one woman who could not endure the odour of her mother's body. She had no problem cuddling in her father's arms, or with other people, but the smell of her mother's body made her sick to her stomach. She still remembers the guilt she felt during her mother's funeral - guilt that she had never been able to show the affection she wanted to give to her mother and guilt for being unable to share this problem with her mother. Through it all, there was the intense feeling of grief for all she had missed throughout her life.

Taking time to consider super sensitivity to smell may result in the elimination of the most frustrating of problems. A daycare was having problems with one of its children. The child knew how to put on his shoes, and usually did so when asked, except when he arrived at the daycare. The staff determined that the behaviour was the result of separation anxiety from his mother, which they felt should gradually subside over time. However, years have passed and this behaviour persisted.

As I went through the sensory behaviour exhibited by this boy and mentioned his obvious problems with the sense of smell, the daycare workers all looked at each other and simultaneously said "the diaper pail". It seems that they were expecting this boy to put on and tie his shoes right beside the diaper pail. Giving the boy the opportunity to use the front odour (no diaper pail) rather than the back door completely eliminated the shoe tying problem.

Getting this message through to the staff at the daycare was simple compared to convincing the mother. I had determined that the boy was sensitive to smell because he often had two fingers stuffed up his nose. At one point, when his riding instructor approached, he covered up both his nose and mouth completely with a cupped hand. The mother didn't see this behaviour as a reaction to smell. She was convinced that it was an abnormal and totally unacceptable social behaviour which he had acquired through imitation of another child. She also fully believed that he did it because he realized it aggravated her. She was constantly reminding him to take his fingers out of his nose, and paid little attention to my diagnosis. She was confident there was no way she could feel comfortable with this behaviour.

The last day I was with the family, we were at the daycare together. I was in the kitchen where the cook had been making spicy cookies and the cleaning lady was busy scrubbing with a very strong Pine Sol solution. As I opened the swinging door, these odours wafted into the next room with me. The mother was helping her son put on his jacket and as the smells hit him, his fingers went straight up into his nostrils. How powerful a demonstration. From then on, the mother concentrated on the environment as a clue to her son's behaviour.

As caregivers, we have to be aware that smell may be the cause of a lot of the agitation. It is important to try and eliminate as much stress in this area as possible. If something smells bad to us, it likely is even more obnoxious to the individual with autism. Most of the time, we may not even be aware there is an odour. Habituation is the ability to switch off smells so they are no longer registered. This is not the blocking of sensory input, which we have mentioned before, but instead is the automatic blocking of a recurring odour or other sensation to which we have no need to respond. Our normal household odours are a good example of habituation. It is only when you walk in the door that you notice them. The longer you stay, the less you smell them.

As we have mentioned in previous chapters, habituation responses for individuals with autism have been measured. Autistic subjects do not habituate as readily as "normal subjects".[202] If one considers the lack of habituation and the high acuity to odour, one may be able to explain why people with autism have so much trouble with change. The increased time it takes to habituate means that the odours in a new environment will be noticeable for longer periods of time, leading to more anxiety. Constantly changing environments become extremely stressful.

Sometimes it is impossible to eliminate an odour. I was driving down the road with one of my clients when we came to an area where there was a heavy petroleum smell. He began to show signs of agitation by flipping his fingers, squirming in his seat and tapping his feet. Instead of concerning myself with these behaviours, I concentrated on the environment. I turned to him and said "My that's an awful smell, isn't it? I do hope that we get through it soon." He glanced at me and relaxed. The fact that the smell was apparent to me as well as to him and that I shared his feelings of discomfort obviously offered him solace.

Individuals with Autism Say ...

> ..."You liked the smell of certain foods, and hated the smell of others, Georgie, but what about people? And animals? How did they smell?" She looked sheepish. "I still have trouble with that," she said. "Dogs and cats. And smells like deodorant and after-shave lotion, they smell so strong to me I can't stand it, and perfume drives me nuts. I can't understand why people wear perfume, and I can smell hand lotion from the next room."[203]

> According to Jerry, his childhood experience could be summarized as consisting of two predominant experiential states, confusion and terror ... living in a frightening world presenting painful stimuli that could not be mastered. Noises were unbearably loud; smells overpowering.[204]

> Albert's memory for detail is striking, "I remember when I was 1 year old I went to Nashville, the air sometimes smelled like firewood. I remember hearing music, it bugged me a lot." Albert continued, "I knew I was in a different place, I woke up and smelled the air it was like a whole bunch of old buildings."…. Albert claims he does not understand why he cannot maintain a friendship. When asked what he usually discusses with his classmates, he replies, "Wind and different smells in the environment."[205]

Indications of Sensitivity to Odour

Watch for:

- Stopping up nostrils with the fingers, covering the nose with the hand or constantly waving one's hand in front of the mouth and nose area.

- Agitation in an environment that has a noticeable smell. The smell may be noxious or sweet.

- Breathing through the mouth rather than the nose.

The high level of smell for individuals with autism means that they are able to detect many smells we cannot. It also means that the smells we deal with on a regular basis are likely very overwhelming to them. Increased agitation without an observable reason may result from an annoying odour.

Human odours may be strong and overwhelming. These may change throughout the day and are different for each individual. Masking our natural human smell with perfume and deodorant may create combinations that are overwhelming to these children.

Menstruation causes its own unique odour. Women may notice increased difficulties with a child during this period of time.

Some children with autism are able to smell over great distances, whereas we cannot.

The smell of their own urine and bowel movements may be overpowering. They may refuse to go to the bathroom until they can no longer restrain themselves. It may lead to constipation problems. On the other hand, they may use the smell of bowel movements to over stimulate, and cut out the senses, by smearing their excrement.

Being close to people is a problem. Even if they do not have physical contact with them, their body odour may be overpowering.

There may be an aversion to foods that have a strong or different odour.

Certain environments may be a problem -- farms, petting zoos, areas with a heavy petroleum smell, and fish stores. Refusal to go into a certain area, or distress when going towards something, may well indicate a sensitivity in this area.

Pet smells may be too much for the child.

Memories of odours may also be a problem. One child returned from a school field trip talking about pigs which continued on for several weeks. Only when he was older was he able to share with his parents that it was the smell of the pigs that affected him so.

The use of various alcohol products may cause people to emit a unique odour. An individual with autism may try to avoid a person who has been drinking. I have noticed this reaction after a group of us shared a bottle of wine.

Method of Care

Do not concentrate on the behaviour, concentrate on the environment. Never discipline individuals with autism for plugging their nostrils with their fingers. They are doing so as a measure of protection, not to irritate anyone, or because it is bad manners.

Keep Kleenex on hand and offer them to the person with autism often, since they may touch their noses much more than we do.

Be aware that odour may be a problem, even if we do not notice it.

If there is a slightly noxious odour in the environment, realize that the individual with autism will likely find it more irritating than we do. Respond to any resulting agitation by talking about it.

Keep perfumed products in our environment at a minimum. They may smell nice to us, but may be overpowering to those with autism. Combinations of different scents can also cause problems.

Any person working with people with autism should keep the use of perfumed products to a minimum. Again this especially applies to a mixture of different smells. If we take the time to count the different body products we use each day, which may contain different perfumes, we can recognize how big a problem it can be. Soap, shampoo, conditioners, hand and body lotions, makeup, deodorant, colognes or perfumes, toothpaste, mouthwash, as well as laundry products which perfume our clothes, are often used daily by most of us, with little or no thought of how any of them smell, or affect the way we smell.

Keep the environment clean and dry. Damp areas may lead to mustiness that we may not notice, but may bother individuals with autism.

While doing laundry, use scent-free products. This includes the softeners, as well as the detergents. Borax is an excellent product for removing odours (anything from urine to perfume) and makes clothes fresh without any scent. It is also environmentally friendly.

Be cautious using face cloths to wash the face. The odour may be unbearable if the cloth has been washed in a perfumed detergent. It may smell stale if it has been used once and left to dry.[206]

Bath time may be affected by odour in many different ways.

Some individuals with autism will use their feces as a way to over stimulate themselves and thus cut out stimulation. Other strong scents may be used as a reward system to eliminate this behaviour.

Other individuals with autism have been found to stimulate themselves on the scratch and sniff type stickers used as rewards, or on the perfumed inks of scented pens. This is another method of overwhelming their systems in order to cut out stimulation. Access to these products should be limited.

An idea that helps some people with odour sensitivity is to apply a strong smelling ointment, which they enjoy (eucalyptus is a choice many make), to their upper lip. The proximity of this smell blocks other smells from the environment. This allows them to be in environments with obnoxious or too many different odours without a build-up of anxiety.

Conclusion

Hyper smell is probably the hardest of the senses for us to comprehend and recognize. We often take no notice of odours and therefore the abnormal behaviour seems to happen for no reason.

The professional world is willing to go to some extreme lengths to reveal the problem of hyper smell as revealed in a case study by Dr. Delacato.[207] He recognized the behaviour of fanning the face as an indication that the boy perhaps had a problem with hyper acuity to odour. The boy seemed intrigued with the smoke coming from the doctor's cigarette. In order to make contact, the doctor blew a stream of smoke in the boy's face. Their eyes met, the boy smiled faintly and proceeded to vomit all over the office rug.

Somehow, I feel there are ways we need to be more cautious and caring with those who have autism. Pushing them to the limits of nausea is neither empathetic or ethical. Trying to understand, although perhaps frustrating is, in the long run, the proper method of care.

198 Diane Ackerman, *The Natural History of the Senses* (New York: Random House, 1990) p. 10.

199 Donald McBurney and Virginia Collings, *Introduction to Sensation/ Perception* Second Edition (Englewood Cliffs, New Jersey: Prentice-Hall Inc. 1984) pp. 87-88.

200 Diane Ackerman, p. 5.

201 T. G. R. Bower, *The Perceptual World of the Child* (Cambridge, Massachusetts: Harvard University Press, 1980) p. 19.

202 Karl Reichelt, G. Saelid, T. Lindback, & J. Boler, "Childhood Autism, a complex disorder," *Biological Psychiatry* (Vol. 21, 1986) pp. 1279-1290.

203 Annabel Stehli, *The Sound of a Miracle* (New York: Doubleday, 1991) p. 187.

204 J. Bemporad, "Adult recollections of a formerly autistic child," *Journal of Autism and Developmental Disorders* (Vol. 9, no. 2, 1979) p. 192.

205 Laura Cesaroni and Malcolm Garber, "Exploring the experience of autism through firsthand accounts," *Journal of Autism and Developmental Disorders* (Vol. 21, no. 3, 1991) pp. 307 and 310.

206 Carl Delacato, *The Ultimate Stranger The Autistic Child* (Novato, California: Academic Publications, 1974) p. 122.

207 Carl Delacato, p. 16-17.

Chapter Seven

Taste

Taste is likely the most confusing of the senses when dealing with an individual with autism as a child's reaction to the food he is served may have absolutely nothing at all to do with the actual taste of that food. However, a healthy diet is important in building and maintaining a strong body, and, therefore, we must not only take this sense into consideration, but be very aware of the many different problems with diet. This chapter will focus more on diet as a whole, rather than on taste as a separate sense.

Accounts by parents note the abnormal eating and drinking habits of their children with autism. For example:

> Ken is epileptic and is on Tegretol tablets. He attends a clinic for epileptics. He also suffered from constipation as a baby, but this is carefully monitored at the institution, and appears to have been corrected. He also drinks a lot more liquid than the rest of the family and has been known, on his weekly home visits, to take the dog's bowl and help himself to water from our dam. He has also been known to get water from our toilet with a jug ... eating remains a problem. Ken only eats certain foods, while Sam eats extremely slowly and must chew everything to a pulp before he will swallow it.[208]

Other parents have noted the extreme desire for salt and the need to clear the home of all toxic substances in order to protect their child from poisoning.[209] An obsessive behaviour of licking human skin or objects should be recognized as an extreme desire and effective method to obtain salt.

Individuals with Autism Say ...

> I remember sitting at the table and hating dinner time - staring at my food knowing that it would make me gag if I tried to eat it and that would make my parents mad. Other people constantly teased me about how I ate my food. Kids are supposed to like chocolate, whipped cream and maple syrup; I didn't. I don't like vegetables either. Cheese, creams, sauces, casseroles, salads - nothing. I hate being invited out or over to eat - it's never how I like to eat it. People keep telling me I would grow to like other foods, I'm still waiting. B. Kirby[210]

> There are few foods that I can tolerate eating. Usually the ones I can eat are soft textured. Italian seems to be the limit. Sometimes I think it is a wonder that I am still alive." Thomas McKean[211]

> I had a big problem with food. I liked to eat things that were bland and uncomplicated. My favourite foods were cereal - dry, not with milk - bread, pancakes, macaroni and spaghetti, potatoes and milk. Because these were the foods I ate early in life, I found them comforting and soothing. I didn't want to try anything new.

> I was supersensitive to the texture of food, and I had to touch everything with my fingers to see how it felt before I put it in my mouth. I really hated it when food had things mixed with it, like noodles with vegetables or bread with fillings to make sandwiches. I could never, never put any of it into my mouth. I knew that if I did I would get violently sick.

Once when I was very small, I tried to eat a banana for my grandmother, but I couldn't do it. So, from then on, I refused to eat any of the other fruits. I wanted to eat the things I was used to; the others were very threatening to me. When Mom tried to get me to eat something new I got very angry with her - I knew what I wanted! Sean Barron[212]

It is very difficult to separate the sense of acute taste from problems that occur due to the sense of smell, touch, hearing, and, sometimes, even sight. As a caregiver, one must remember to be very aware that eating problems may be linked to one or all of the senses. If a child has eating problems, it is important to take all the senses into account. Note that there are many situations mentioned throughout the methods of care in the previous chapters that involve meals.

The sense of taste may well have nothing to do with the inability of a person to digest a certain food. When one works closely with those who have autism, one can recognize certain problems in regard to certain foods. I have mentioned these both in the general observations and method as well as in a special section on Allergies at the end of the chapter.

Indications of Diet Sensitivities

Watch for:

- The refusal to eat certain foods.
- An insistence on eating only a limited number of foods.

There is often stubborn resistance to trying out new foods. Babies seem to have difficulties progressing from a liquid diet to one that includes solids. This likely indicates a problem with texture, rather than with taste.

At times, individuals with autism seem willing to eat or drink anything. They appear to have no sense of taste.

There may be a lack of interest in or refusal to eat wheat products such as bread, or signs of difficulty in digesting wheat products (constipation or bloated stomach). Medical practitioners have noticed that bowel movements may smell like those of people with celiac disease. Yet, when tested, individuals with autism do not show the same gastrointestinal symptoms.[213]

Digestion problems may also happen when one ingests milk products. Some individuals may refuse to eat or drink milk products. Others may have an abnormal craving for milk.

There is usually a lack of interest in sweets.

Some individuals with autism seem to love the taste of salt and may have a tendency to crave salty food. Those who have autism may also lick people's skin and objects to satisfy their craving for salt.

They often exist on limited diets and yet remain healthy.

They drink an excessive amount of water and will go to extremes to get it. These extremes may well be the result of the tendency to limit the amount of fluids allowed individuals who are not toilet trained. This practice does far more harm than good.

An abrupt change in behaviour may occur within a certain time frame after eating certain foods.

Garlic seemed to result in agitation with three young men the day after it was used in meals. For some people, garlic causes headaches. This may well have been happening to the people with whom we were working.

Watch for adverse reactions to some antibiotics, and to the fillers in certain medications. For example, a young lad I worked with reacted with extreme head banging shortly after taking a generic form of ativan. Later we noticed that he started head banging after taking antibiotic pills for an ear infection. Switching to a liquid form of antibiotic eliminated this adverse reaction.

Method of Care

Refusal to eat wheat or milk products should be respected. On the other hand, craving a dietary item such as wheat or milk may also indicate intolerance to the substance that is craved.

A high protein diet seems to cut down the level of agitation. While working with autistic individuals, I have noticed an easy acceptance and enjoyment of bean and lentil dishes.

Never limit liquid intake; their bodies need it. One man states that dehydration is his most common cause of headaches and clouded thinking.

Vitamin B6 and Magnesium supplements seem to help.[214]

Keep all poisonous substances locked safely away. If these individuals have blocked out sensation, they may well eat or drink anything.

Eating or drinking foods with an extreme flavour, such as drinking whole bottles of Tabasco sauce at once, may be an attempt to block the sensation of taste.

A fatty, salty diet, especially in the morning, also seems to work well with some individuals with autism

Individuals with autism do not react the same to sedation as do other people. They are often given very high doses of a sedative in order to be put to sleep. Turkey has biochemicals which naturally make us sleepy. If a person with autism is to be undergoing medical treatment or testing which will require sedation, have them eat several turkey meals in advance.[215] The sedation will have a better effect.

One concern we must always be aware of is the inability to feel hunger when one is under considerable stress and blocking out sensation in one way or another. Caregivers must always be aware if individuals with autism are not eating. This is not because they are not hungry, but that they are blocking out their feelings of hunger. This is especially a problem for adults who have moved out and are living on their own. Often they do not notice what they are doing to their bodies by missing meals and health problems can arise. The lack of food will also lead to more stress and often increased levels of frustration and over stimulation. This can often spiral out of control. It is imperative that concerned friends keep an eye on how much people with autism are eating in order to alleviate problems.

Allergies?

Professionals throughout the world have connected the syndrome of autism to the diet of the child. This theory is based on the discovery (using a 24-hour urine analysis) that relatively high levels of biologically active peptides occur in subjects with autism.[216] It is believed that these peptides do not originate in the central nervous system. The incomplete breakdown of protein in the digestive system may be responsible.[217]

Doctors in Norway have taken this theory a step further and developed a gluten and casein free diet. For the last four years, they have tested this diet on a group of 15 individuals with autism.[218] After three years, these children were found to be easier to work with, able to concentrate on tasks, easier to communicate with, less fearful, less agitated, and less sensitive to stimulation. They also expressed emotions more freely and had an increase on IQ test scores.

Other children have gone to doctors who specialize in the field of allergies and have received individualized diets. For one young girl, the new diet is attributed to have produced these results: initiates physical contact with family members, good eye contact, less agitation and repetition, increased play with toys, increased exploration of environment and use of objects, increased sign and verbal communication and potty trained within three months of beginning the new diet.[219]

One child had wheat, corn, and milk eliminated from his diet. Within four days he was more alert and less hyperactive. He also gave up spinning. In five weeks his social behaviour had improved, his nose had stopped running, he was less clumsy and better coordinated. He was learning the alphabet and had begun to read. In time, he graduated from high school with B's and C's and moved on to a Trade School. He is a bit of a loner, but gets along well in school, church and the community.[220]

In other cases, a yeast and sugar free diet has been prescribed when a reaction to mushrooms and yeast were noted. Recurrent ear infections had led to the administration of a lot of antibiotic medicines to these children. The medication led to a recurrent problem with candida (a yeast infection). Nystatin was prescribed to kill the yeast fungus in the digestive tract. The combination of medicine and diet is reported to have decreased the autistic behaviour for two young lads.[221]

Recently, there have been a few reports of problems in breaking down foods high in beta carotene, such as carrots, squashes, sweet potatoes and pumpkins.[222] These do not show up as a problem during allergy tests, but when removed from the diet of a child, improvements in behaviour are noted. The negative reaction is swift, if and when, they are reintroduced. Donna Williams claims that one carrot brings back all her super sensitivities immediately after eating it.[223] I find it interesting to note that we have always been told that eating carrots improves eyesight. Perhaps some old wives' tales are true.

The most exciting response to a change of diet that I have discovered is that with Donna Williams.[224] Donna has been on a diet which removed two phenolic compounds from what she eats; gallic acid and malvin. It is believed that she has an intolerance to these substances. Her diet is based on the work of Dr. Abram Ber of Phoenix, Arizona.

I was personally with Donna both before and after she started the diet. It radically changed her life. It's effects are very noticeable. Donna claims that the super sensitivities she has experienced all her life have been eliminated by this diet and that she is now able to experience the environment in much the same way as do you or I.

Most of the foods we eat and the liquids we drink contain either gallic acid or malvin, so Donna is on a very limited quantity of foods. It is recommended that a person only stick to this diet short-term, but the dramatic change in her life has made it difficult for Donna to resume eating the things that make her super sensitivities return. While dieting she ate only millet, buckwheat, oats, rice and 100% rye as grains; pork, rabbit, duck and fish (except tuna, salmon or halibut) as meats; broccoli, turnip, cauliflower, asparagus, artichoke and sweet potato as vegetables; papaya as a fruit; sesame, sunflower and safflower as oils; peanut butter and tahini as spreads; ryvitas (sesame), rice cakes, oat cakes and rice crackers as crackers; and rice milk, hazelnut milk, brazil nut milk, nettle, dandelion and chamomile teas as beverages.

Would this diet work for anyone else but Donna? Who knows until more research is done in this area? It may be a totally individual case. However, it is a very strong indication that what we eat does affect how well our senses work.

These are a few examples of success stories when diet was changed for children with autism. As with any other treatment, failures have gone unrecorded. The success can be attributed to the biochemicals produced in the brain and the need for adequate nutrients to produce these biochemicals. I fully believe that diet is the one area upon which more research should focus.

The brain uses various amino acids to manufacture the neurotransmitters used to link neurons in the transfer of signals throughout the nervous system.[225] These amino acids come into the body through our diet and are transported to the brain via the bloodstream. The amount of neurotransmitters used when signals are sent affects the strength of the signal. A shortage of the amino acid to produce the neurotransmitters should indicate that less stimulation would occur. Examples of the biochemicals which are produced from amino acids include serotonin, acettylcholine, dopamine, norepinephrine and pinephrine. It is interesting to note that the neurotransmitters - serotonin, dopamine, and norepinephrine - have all been found in higher than normal levels in subjects with autism.[226]

As parents or caregivers, we should consider the diet of our children and how it may contribute to their problems. Since this book cannot go into all the details, I would suggest you contact a local allergy specialist if you believe your child may be suffering in this area.[227] Specialists around the world have been concentrating on the role of diet with children who have learning difficulties or who are very hyperactive. It may be advisable to check out literature from this field of study, or search for this type of specialist.

If you are interested in more information on the gluten and casein free diets, there is abundant information and discussion of this topic on the Internet.[228]

Conclusion

In my work with people with autism, I have found that they seem to know what they want when it comes to food and drink. No matter how bizarre and limited these diets appear, they do not seem to result in any major health problems. Individuals with autism also seem to realize which foods make them feel better.

One young boy went on a vacation with his family when he was about eight years old. At the hotel where they were staying, the family was served a breakfast of sausages and fries every morning. His parents found it a greasy and salty meal, not one they enjoyed, or felt good about. The son claimed that these meals made him feel calm and able to cope throughout each day in a way he had never felt before. He has insisted on eating this breakfast every day for the last fourteen years. He is doing well, as he has just completed a four year degree at college and is now employed.

It is interesting to note that a diet rich in fat was developed by the John Hopkins Medical Centre and the Mayo Clinic to decrease the potential for seizures in the brain.[229] The diet was developed in 1927 and has been used successfully as a treatment measure for the last forty years. However, it's popularity declined with the development of anticonvulsant drugs, until lately. It is now becoming popular as an alternative to drugs for children who suffer seizures.

This "high-fat diet produces ketosis, or ketones, in the blood, which are breakdown products of fat. This produces acidosis in the blood which also finds its way to the fluid surrounding the brain. Brain fluid with more acid in it decreases the potential for having seizures by decreasing the electrical excitability in the brain."[230] Does the diet chosen by the young man with autism work in the same way? Only extensive research in the future will let us know for sure.

I do feel it is important to stimulate these children by exposing them to different foods. However, as a caregiver, I do not believe that a varied diet is the most important factor when it comes to food. Respect for personal individual choice and feelings seems far more important than restricting them to a certain diet.

208 Personal correspondence from a parent of twins who have autism.

209 A. Lovell, *In a Summer Garment: The experience of an Autistic Child* (London: Secker and Warburg, 1978) p. 21.

210 "What the DSM-IV means to me...", from the Internet, March 1996, address: http://www.udel.edu/bkirby/asperger/asmeansl.html.

211 Thomas McKean, " An alternate look at autistic perceptions," in *A World of Options* Conference proceedings, (Toronto: Autism Society of America and Autism Society Canada, July, 1993) p. 30.

212 Judy Barron and Sean Barron, *There's a Boy in Here* (New York: Simon and Schuster, 1992) p. 96.

213 Bernard Rimland, Megavitamins, Hypoglycemia and Food Intolerances as Related to Autism [Presentation] (Flint, Michigan: National Society for Autistic Children, 1972) p. 9.

214 Bernard Rimland, E. Callaway, and P. Dreyfus, "The effect of high doses of vitamin B6 on autistic children: a double blind crossover study," *American Journal of Psychiatry* (Vol. 135, no. 4, 1978) pp. 472-475.

215 Nancy Brehm, personal communication.

216 Paul Shattock, "Protein, peptides and problems in autism," in *Proceedings from Therapeutic Approaches to Autism: research and Practice Conference* (Durham: Autism Research Unit and the National Society of Autism, Great Britain, 1991) p. 176.

217 Ann-Mari Knivsberg, Kristi Wiig, Gunnar Lind, Magne Nodland and Karl, L. Reichelt, " Dietary intervention in autistic syndromes," *Brain Dysfunction* (Vol. 3, 1990) p. 315-316.

218 Ann-Mari Knivsberg, Magnus Nodland and Karl Reichelt, "Gluten and/or casein free diets as treatment," in *Proceedings from the Therapeutic Approaches to Autism: Research and Practice Conference* (Durham: Autism Research Unit and The National Autism Society of Great Britain, 1991) p. 165.

219 Donna Calvera, Angela is Coming Home [Handout #32] (San Diego: The Institute of Child Research, 1976) p. 3-4.

220 William Crook and Laura Stevens, *Solving the Problem of Your Hard-To-Raise Child* (New York: Random House, 1987) p. 283.

221 William Crook and Laura Stevens, pp. 285-287.

222 Adair Renning, personal communication.

223 Donna Williams, "Speaks on her life and struggle" (audiotape of presentation at Autism '96 Orlando, FL conference, February 1996) Available through Future Horizons, Inc.

224 Ibid.

225 William Crook and Laura Stevens, pp. 224-225.

226 J. Gerald Young, Mary Ellen Kavanaugh, George Anderson, Bennett Shaywitz and Donald Cohen, "Clinical disorders of autism and associated disorders," Journal of Autism and *Developmental Disorders* (Vol. 12, no. 2, 1982), pp. 148, 153 & 158.

227 For more information on this subject as well as a support group of parents contact Allergy-induced Autism Support and Self-Help Group, c/o Brenda O'Reilly, 3 Palmera Avenue, Calcott, Reading, Berkshire, RG3 7DZ, Great Britain. This group is presently involved in research in the area of enzymes needed for digestion and the differences in an autistic population. Watch for developments in this area.

228 Dianne Woodward: email address: rwoodwardw@|sumc.edu or parlante@aol.com.

229 Chris Zdeb Montgomery, "Sick kids 'reborn' under diet of whipping cream and oil", *The Edmonton Journal* (March 1, 1996) p. B3.

230 Ibid.

Chapter Eight

Social Interaction

A parent related an encounter, between her teenage son and a school mate in a shopping mall, to a group of parents and professionals. As she described the rude behaviour of the school mate towards her son, all of us were filled with a common sense of sadness and futility. A speech language pathologist tried to calm the mother with these words. "Isn't it good that Charles doesn't know what is going on, like we do."

The myth that the autistic population lacks social feelings; so glibly accepted throughout the professional world, is heartrending. Those simple words of comfort may have eased the pain and helplessness of the mother for the moment but the disservice they did her son, and all others with autism, was immeasurable. Individuals with autism do have feelings- very strong feelings. Their lack of understanding of the acceptable behaviours for social competence has absolutely nothing to do with a lack of feeling. As long as we deny them their feelings, they have no opportunity to express themselves and to learn new behaviours which will help them in the area of social interaction.

The importance of friendship in one's everyday existence is one of the prime considerations for every parent of a child with autism. It is a goal that seems impossible to attain. In order to help, our attitudes must go through a series of changes. We must discard the idea that autism means lack of feeling. We have to dispel the myth that lack of feeling is an innate feature of autism or a prime indication of brain dysfunction. We must review the areas of acute sensitivity to stimulation and recognize how the symptoms we accept as an indication of impairment in social interaction, actually reinforce the sensory theory of autism.

As I have mentioned throughout this book, little significance is placed on the sensory reactions of individuals with autism when the condition is diagnosed. The Diagnostic and Statistical Manual of the American Psychiatric Association, fourth edition (DSM-IV) is the current standard of measurement for autism. In order to be labelled autistic one must exhibit:

1. a qualitative impairment in reciprocal social interaction,
2. a qualitative impairment in verbal and non verbal communication and in imaginative activity,
3. a markedly restricted repertoire of activities and interests and
4. onset during infancy or childhood.

Additionally, there should be a delay or abnormal functioning in at least one of the following (with onset prior to age 3 years): social interaction, language as used in social communication, or symbolic or imaginative play. Also, the condition is not better accounted for by the diagnosis of Rett's Disorder or Childhood Disintegrative Disorder.[231]

If the professional world insists on concentrating only on the above symptoms of autism, without any consideration for where the symptoms originate, the plight of individuals with autism will remain critical. In order to understand the impairments we see in social interaction, communication and so on, we must take into consideration the various experiences of an oversensitive infant from the onset of life.

Consider this......A child with autism is born and is tactile sensitive. In other words, he cannot stand to be touched. He is a small infant. Who do we touch more than our newborn infants? He cries because it is painful to be held. What do we do with a crying infant? What is our natural response? We cuddle him, we hold him, and we rock him. In doing so, we inadvertently inflict more pain. The only way to eliminate this pain is to leave him alone.[232] The child learns, at a very young age, not to use the natural method of infant communication because our response to the communication leads to pain. The child learns not to cry for anything. This doesn't mean he is a placid happy baby. I believe it means he is protecting himself from tactile stimulation.

From the very beginning of life, a child with autism may demonstrate an impairment in the natural communication process, an impairment that is not a dysfunction of the brain, but an impairment that is caused directly by tactile sensitivity. This child is forced to find new ways to communicate and to interact with his mother or other caregivers. He withdraws; he stiffens when held or goes absolutely limp. He lies quietly in the crib, making very few demands on anyone.

The whole communication pattern changes for the rest of his life. Feelings are covered up. Social interaction, for this child, will always be different than for normal children. Unless we recognize that tactile sensitivity is present, is causing pain, and respect this fact we will not make effort to develop safe and pleasing ways to interact with the child. Their social skills will continue to be impaired.

If we review some of the common assumptions about autistic behaviour which lead professionals to recognize social impairment, we find more indications of tactile sensitivity. The "failure to assume at any time an anticipatory posture preparatory to being picked up"[233] is one of the main features described as an indication of early social impairment. This was included in the first article on autism by Kanner in 1943 and is noted on behaviour checklists by most parents. Kanner also included another indication of social impairment as the "lack of ability" to adjust one's body to the posture of the person holding him.[234] Are these truly an indication of social impairment, especially an impairment which indicates brain dysfunction?

Why would infants, who do not want to be touched because it hurts, ever assume the anticipatory position to being picked up? They do not want to be picked up! Would it not be more logical for us to assume that the lack of this response indicates a lack of desire to be held? Do they lack the ability to adjust their posture to the person holding them? There is a big difference between the lack of ability and the desire to react in a certain manner. Are not these babies attempting to get through the experience of being held with as little pain as possible? Obviously, these behaviours reveal sensitivity to tactile stimulation, not dysfunction in the brain. What we have is an early adaptation to one's actual experience, as well as the very functional development of protective behaviours, behaviours which tie directly to tactile sensitivity. If we are to help those who have autism, we must not assume that they lack feeling or ability. It is time to recognize the behaviours for what they really represent.

Later in life a child told his mother "I know I should love you but I don't know why." The mother, using natural human behaviour, hugs the child as she tells him she loves him. In this instance we have words and emotions which are supposed to make one feel good. At the same time we are providing a tactile experience that may feel awful to the individual with autism. Remember, some people who have autism describe physical contact as intolerable, overwhelming, excruciating, and unbearable. Is it not safe to assume that they will be confused by this dual message and not be able to really understand what love should feel like? Why would you ever want to love someone if the physical feeling you associate it with is intolerable?

The questions we ought to be asking ourselves are innumerable. Why would a small child interact normally with other children when he is trying to avoid physical contact? For that matter, considering how noisy little children are, why expose oneself to the auditory pain? Where and how do so-called normal people learn their acceptable social behaviours? These behaviours are acquired or learned through interaction with their peers while supervised by adults. Children with autism have been forced to withdraw into a world of their own in order to protect themselves. In this world, the natural lessons of social conduct, which most people learn without any effort, are disregarded. This does not mean that people with autism lack feelings or abilities. It only indicates that they have not had the same chance to learn the lessons. As caregivers, we must provide these lessons. We cannot reach this goal unless we have accepted and understood their actual feelings.

Direct eye contact is considered a prime sign of social awareness in our society while lack of eye contact is another indication of impairment of social interaction, stressed by professionals in the field of autism. As we noted in the visual chapter, the lack of eye contact, on the part of individuals with autism has absolutely nothing to do with social behaviour. I think those who have autism avoid direct eye contact because it is too painful. The use of peripheral vision provoked by acute sensitivity means that the person with autism may well be looking at our eyes when we do not realize it. Until we accept this reality, and stop insisting on eye contact as a means to communicate and socially interact, it is we, the caregivers, who are stuck.

Another indication of social impairment is the lack of facial expression. Again, we have to consider the use of peripheral vision in order to protect one's eyes from too much stimulation. Three different social interaction results occur when one uses peripheral vision. First, the ability to make out specific features is limited when one is visually over stimulated; the details are missing. As Dietmar Zoller said in the introduction to his book "people were monsters, forms made out of fat without contours".[235] Secondly, the behaviour of the caregiver is also affected by the behaviour of the individual with autism. If we only react socially by displaying appropriate facial expressions when they are looking directly at us (at which time they are actually looking somewhere else), we don't give them the opportunity to react to, or to learn, the different expressions which designate the different emotions. In the third place, our definition of the situation also affects this "social impairment symptom." Catherine Lord has done a study in which she monitored the faces of her autistic subjects and discovered that they were indeed using appropriate facial expressions,[236] but only when they were looking off to the side of the person with whom they were interacting.

Another aspect of sensory stimulation which creates problems in the area of social interaction is sound. If individuals cannot decipher the conversation of the people who are interacting with them, they will not be able to respond in an acceptable manner. They may not be able to understand what is going on.

Robbie's father would take him to the local McDonald's restaurant for supper. After they finished eating, Robbie would join the group of children in the play area of the restaurant. One day, the group was involved in a game of follow the leader, and Robbie actively took part as a follower. The leader suddenly called out "everyone go the opposite direction." All the children turned around and went the other way. Robbie reacted in confusion and retreated from the game with a very dejected look on his face.

We have to realize that the problem this child encountered was that he could not decipher what the leader said because it was too loud. Robbie felt totally left out of the group. If the instructions had been given to him quietly, by another child, he could have been part of the whole game. Perhaps an adult could have shared this information with the child, letting him know exactly what had been said without making a big deal about the fact the child could not decipher it. The group of children did not choose to reject Robbie. In fact, they had no more idea of what happened than he did. As long as Robbie understands this, he can develop socially. If he felt that they were rejecting him (which he obviously did by the look on his face), and if he had no idea why, he cannot grow in a healthy social manner. He may well adopt some pretty "weird" behaviour patterns to compensate as he attempts to be part of his peer group. Naturally, this will only lead to more rejection.

If we do not provide a sense of security and freedom from anxiety for those who have autism, little we attempt to accomplish in the areas of social interaction will be worthwhile As long as they need to be in control, and on the alert, in order to protect themselves, we will not be able to get through to them. Self-protection will always take precedence over any social interaction.

Individuals with autism rarely understand just how they are different from the normal population. This does not mean they do not realize they are different and do not care. They are often as unaware of the fact that they see, hear, and smell more acutely than we do, as we are to their experiences. They often believe that we "normal" people have the same experiences and that we are somehow able to cope better. For example, we can look at the words of Sean Barron as found in the book, *There's a Boy in Here*. "All I wanted was to be like the other kids my age. It felt as if I was weird and strange on the outside, but inside I wasn't like that. The inside person wanted to get out and break free of all the behaviours that I was a slave to and couldn't stop."[237]

Donna Williams, as an adult, questions our differences:

How can they sit in this room?, I wondered. Perhaps it was me? Perhaps their volume and brightness control didn't go up like mine did. Perhaps their maker set their switches and that was that. Perhaps their switches didn't slip out of tune every time there was something new to take in. Awesome.[238]

Explaining the extreme sensitivity to stimulation is the first method we can use with those who have autism to allow them to come to terms with the differences they perceive. Accepting the need for protective behaviours is the next step. These behaviours develop at a very young age and become habitual. In other words, the individual often becomes oblivious, not only to the actions, but often to the reasons these behaviours take place.

On the other hand, peers in the social community are not oblivious to behaviours which are considered strange or bizarre and react accordingly. The individual is shunned, mocked, or bullied. This cruel behaviour does not go unheeded by the individual with autism. As Thomas McKean says, "Of course it hurt, what do you think? I am a human being."[239] Throughout his autobiography, Sean Barron vividly describes the torment of many incidents of cruelty and teasing during his years at school.[240] Individuals with autism may experience a real lack of understanding of social situations. This plight is often shared with parents and caregivers by verbal individuals. The lack of understanding does not mean at any time that the pain of rejection, mockery and cruelty is not felt deeply. It only means that these people do not know what to do about it. We must realize that they do not understand why their peers are reacting to them in this way. They also lack the understanding how to change their own behaviour to fit the pattern of those who are so-called "socially correct."

Children can be very cruel to anyone who is different. A difference in skin colour, nationality, dress code, or in the ability/disability to live in our world can all result in teasing, rejection, and cruelty. Just being the new kid on the block or perhaps being interested in astrology instead of baseball can produce these reactions. Minor health problems such as asthma or eczema, to extreme ones such as cerebral palsy or paralysis, can also provoke these cruelties. The extreme protective behaviours of individuals with autism are especially disturbing to those who see themselves as “normal”, and result not only in social rejection by children, but also by adults. We, as caregivers, have to realize that it is not the individuals with autism who are at fault, but rather that normal children need to learn to be more compassionate and accepting. Explaining the differences in sensory experience to these children makes it easier for them to understand the strange behaviours of autism. Showing them safe ways to interact with individuals with autism allows everyone to partake in meaningful social interaction. Ignoring the cruel rejections and allowing them to continue means that we are exposing our children with autism to severe degrees of emotional pain.

In *Autism: a Personal Account* we read:

I hated school. The teachers pretended to be understanding but were not. I was frightened of the girls and boys, the teachers and everything else. I was frightened of the toilets and you had to ask to use them which I was not able to do, also I was never sure when I wanted to go to the toilet anyway and the teachers got fed up with having to take me to the nurse to change me. It was mainly the women that were horrible, the men were a bit nicer. When I was at school I was kicked, hit, pushed over and made fun of by the other children.[241]

The young woman's experiences were so deeply felt she goes as far as to offer this advice, "Parents of autistic children should never think of sending their children to ordinary schools, because the suffering will far outweigh any of the benefits achieved."[242]

Another account of the experience of education is included in *Adult Recollections of a Formerly Autistic Child.* "Elementary school was remembered as a horrifying experience. The classroom was total confusion and he always felt he would go to pieces."[243]

Isolating these children from the world and denying them an education is certainly not the answer. We must recognize that when a person lives in a world dominated by fear and pain, their behaviour and development focuses on protection, not interaction with other members of the species. If we do not take the time to protect those who have autism from overwhelming stimulation, they will be forced to protect themselves. In their world of safety, created by the production of endorphins, these children will not be aware of the lessons of socialization, much less be able to learn them. As they get older, social interplay may become obvious to them. They do not have any real understanding of how to interact because they have never had a real opportunity to learn the methods. Consequently, the teenage years often become the lonely years.

> Jerry's memories of his early life were extremely painful. In childhood, he was simply afraid of human contact; in adolescence, he desired some sort of relationship while the original fear remained unabated. As a teenager, Jerry witnessed other youngsters enjoying camaraderie and social activities and wanted to be included but was too afraid to make a really persistent effort. He would sporadically try to be with peers but quickly retreated to the safety of his own home when others did not treat him as he wished. Again, he simply had no idea of how to go about making interpersonal contact, so that the realistic rejections he suffered added to the distorted expectations of injury that he anticipated.[244]

The individual with autism may well appear not to have any feelings in this regard, as in his own world there are no feelings. That does not mean that those who have autism are unable to feel or have some sort of dysfunction in the brain so they do not feel. It only means that for a time their feelings may be shut off. By providing safe environments in which the need for protection can be ignored, the individual with autism can be free to socialize and to learn social patterns of behaviour like any other human being.

In the meantime, never forget that individuals with autism do have feelings and that these feelings are as important to them as our feelings are to each of us. Denying them their feelings is as cruel and unfeeling as the rejection by their peers because they are different. Loneliness is a big factor in their lives. If we genuinely care, we will take the time to consider the reasons behind their differences and then accept them as unique human beings who are as special as anyone else.

Not only do individuals with autism have their own feelings, they also have the ability to recognize that other people have feelings. When they are not lost in a world of their own, they will try to respect the feelings of others whenever possible. A young woman was invited to attend a banquet in honour of people with disabilities as a representative of the National Autistic Society. The country's president was the guest speaker at the banquet, and when his speech was over everyone rushed forward for the chance to meet the leader of their country. The young woman hesitated and then turned to her mother. "You do understand I can't be part of that." she said. "It's all right," said her mother, who realized that the closeness of the crowd would be much more than her daughter could bear. Then the young girl apologized. "I'm sorry that I have disappointed you." It was a moment this mother will never forget. Her daughter had actually realized that the mother would have been proud to watch her child greet the p`resident. By allowing the young woman the right to her own feelings, the mother had also allowed her daughter the freedom to share her knowledge of her mother's feelings.

Another young lad ran away from his group home in the Rocky Mountains along with two other residents. As a native, who had grown up in the wilderness, he seemed fearless on his own and had often disappeared for days on end. During their first night on the run, the howling of the coyotes terrified his companions. This boy chose to lead them back to the group home on his own, rather than subject them to another night in the wilderness. He was willing to give up his freedom to give them peace of mind.

As well as having the ability to recognize the feelings of other people, individuals with autism have an intuition of how people feel about them. They know if you are treating them as if they are retarded or incapable,[245] and they will react accordingly.

They also may sense how people feel about themselves and seem to have an incredible ability to zero in on the one behaviour which will annoy an individual caregiver the most.[246] A different behaviour will be used to frustrate another caregiver. By making the attempt to understand those who have autism and to really care for them as they are, we give them the opportunity to interact with us without the use of protective behaviours.

Their intuition gives them a window on the feelings of those around them. This is a window they are unable to close, or to ignore. When we, who are working closely with them, feel angry, frustrated, fearful or stressed out, our feelings often overwhelm them and result in the need for protective behaviours. One day, Sharisa Kochmeister was driving with her father, who was terribly upset about a situation in his life which had nothing to do with his daughter. As her behaviours escalated, he realized that she was in trouble and asked what was wrong. She explained that his strong negative feelings were causing her to react in this way.[247] This is not an uncommon situation for people with autism.

Individuals with Autism Say ...

> Autism means having to watch how I feel every second that I am awake. Autism means having challenge when I leave the room fearing that others will say unkind things about me to other people. Autism means being dateless on weekends as well as constant loneliness, only watching TV on Saturday night. Autism means not being able to fit in on social peer relations. However, autism in my case, means that I have a calendar memory for birthdays, being articulate and having skills. I, all in all, would rather be autistic, than normal.[248]
>
> "I'll miss you, Temple." She walked quickly to my side and kissed my cheek. I ached to be enfolded in her arms, but how could she know? I stood rigid as a pole trapped by the approach/avoidance syndrome of autism. I drew back from her kiss, not able to endure tactile stimulation, not even loving, tactile stimulation.[249]
>
> Today, I still prefer to work on my computer or with electronics rather than socialize. I take a magazine to read with me to all social events that I can't get out of. You have to compromise if you're going to have any friends at all. I have managed to finally develop some friendships. It was very difficult in my teens and twenties, but it's easier now. Another good thing that helped with friendships, is that I got my friend a friend. They go to social events together and I'm not made to go. E-mail and the Internet have been a great way for me to make friends.
>
> People seem to have a tendency of placing their needs and social desires on me. They are afraid I'm bored and would enjoy doing the same things that they do. They continue to think that I need to be with people to be happy. I try to assure them that I'm very happy doing just what I'm doing. Most of the time, I get the impression that what they want to say is, "if you like me enough, you'd come to my party..." etc. [250]

Method of Care

People with autism definitely have a delayed level of social development, but they need not withdraw from the world. If we allow it, they actively attempt to interact with their normal counterparts as long as they feel safe and secure enough in their environment. Situations must be developed in which they can interact without fear at a level within their sensory capabilities.

For those of us who work with individuals with autism, the realization that they do not choose to be an active part of social situations may tie directly to the fear and pain of being touched, of loud noises, of overpowering smells, as well as confusion in trying to decipher messages that are too loud, rather than a disability in the area of social interaction. We must be creative in ways to counteract these problems. Individuals who are not allowed to develop socially as children are very, very lonely people, whether or not they have autism.

It is important to provide excellent social situations for interaction in daycare, with baby-sitters, grandparents, the family and friends. As well, give them the opportunity to be alone and in charge of themselves. By adding an understanding of their sensory acuity, and the environment they are part of, these situations will become even more beneficial.

On the other hand, be aware that many people who have autism are not capable of interacting for long periods of time without becoming overstressed. Be aware that more people, more noise, and increased levels of stimulation will provide more arousal. They will need 'time outs' to calm down and relax if visits last for hours. It is best to arrange short visits and outings for young children. As they get older, they will likely be able to cope with more stimulation, and their stress levels will likely decrease, but too much stimulation will still cause problems. As an adult, Sara Miller has difficulty dealing with social situations in which more than four people are involved.[251] Providing a safe area for individuals with autism to retreat to at any age level is beneficial.

Be aware of social standards we force on people because of our own ideas, not because they will make a big difference to the person involved. Appropriate clothing is an excellent example of expectations we may have that do more harm than good. Insisting that someone wear a watch, ring or necklace because we feel it will produce a more normal looking individual, has little benefit if the tactile experience is so negative that the individual with autism can only concentrate on what he or she is wearing. The same goes for rigid collars and ties or scratchy materials such as starched ruffles and lace.

Talking to individuals with autism about their super abilities is of prime importance. They may not realize that other people do not hear, see, feel, taste and smell like they do, any more than we appreciate exactly what they are feeling. The realization of how they are different will make it possible for them to deal with life much more effectively. It also must be stressed that these differences are not bad or stupid. Everyone has differences; everyone is unique in his or her own way. Acceptance of these differences is what makes us a caring human race.

However, we must realize that they will likely require more solitude than other people throughout their lives. They will probably never be the `life of the party' and will always prefer to spend a certain amount of time alone. In order to give them the best opportunity to fit in with their peers, we must respect their unique feelings and provide them with social opportunities in a safe, yet stimulating environment.

We must also realize that there are going to be places and times when they will be over stimulated and may need to use protective behaviours to deal with the situation. Respecting this need is very important. Since the behaviours may not be socially acceptable, it may be wise to suggest that the individual with autism carry out these activities in private. If that is not possible, it may be kinder to explain the reasons for the behaviours to the other people who are present.

Always be aware of your own feelings when working with someone with autism, and realize that the person you are working with may have the intuition to feel what you are feeling, whether it be negative thoughts about themselves, or extreme stress and frustration about something that has nothing to do with them. Their behaviour will be affected by your feelings. The best advice is to be calm and serene at all times when working with people with autism, but realize that this is not a common human ability. If you are upset, share these feelings with them so that they are able to cope with your feelings more effectively. Sharing our feelings also provides role models and the freedom to learn to share their own.

If we do not take the time to understand the real feelings of the people we are working with, even our best attempts to help may end up leading to confusion and frustration. For example, Sara Miller shares this story:

> Many years ago (pre-diagnosis), my husband was trying to teach me to not be so self-conscious, or concerned about what others thought. He used the metaphor of The Duck: "let their comments run off your back like water runs off a duck's back." So he would say "Be like a duck" whenever I was obviously nervous or upset about something. However, my visual picture of

> The Duck was calm to the outside world, but paddling like hell under the surface, so when he said to be like a duck, I felt I was already like a duck.[252]

Sara interpreted her husband's supportive message as "to not let others know how nervous or upset I was." This denial of actual feelings and the attempts to keep them hidden will naturally lead to higher levels of stress and anxiety while interacting with other people.

However, if we accept that the physiological makeup of people with autism is different and that they are reacting more severely within their bodies, we can share an empathy for their actual state. By sharing this information with them, we also give them the chance to realize they are different in this way and, more so, that there is nothing to be ashamed of. Then the goal "to not let others know how nervous and upset one is" can focus on the relationship between people, rather than on guilt or shame. The actual feelings of the individual with autism can be hidden so as not to affect the other person negatively and they can be proud of this accomplishment, or they can be honest and open and admit they are nervous and anxious and that it has very little to do with the other person in the interaction. This frees the person with autism to form real and meaningful relationships with other people.

Because they are immersed in protecting themselves from over stimulation and are often nonverbal, one of the interesting things that happens to children with autism is they miss out completely on the " WHY?" period of life. Typical preschoolers bombard everyone they spend time with the "why" questions, and adults spend hours unconsciously teaching these small children about life. However, we don't take the time to answer those same questions if they are not asked. For the nonverbal child with autism, the questions are as much a part of their life as for any other child, but they do go unasked and unanswered. How much of our social interaction lessons are learned during this period of life, I am not certain. However, I do believe that the "why" questions are very necessary to each and every one of us as a social human being.

The differences in perception, the missed lessons, and the different experiences in life mean that people with autism often communicate with us in ways that we do not quite understand. Problems of communication are discussed by Wally Wojtowicz, Jr. in a letter to his friend Jenny:

> Dad and I sometimes play a word game reminiscent at times of Scrabble. The players take turns scrambling a word and it is up to the other player to make a word out of the scrambled letters. The new word must appear in the dictionary and at times more than one word can be made from different sequences of letters. An example would be: What word or words can you make from these letters: A-C-T?
>
> The two words that can be made are cat and act. In each case, the original three letters are used and the words are found in the dictionary. In retrospect, I think that reordering the letters as new words is as close in practice as anything comes to show a non-autistic person how I think and put the pieces of reality together to make a sensory history of an event I have experienced. I add and subtract, and reorder sensory experiences to find that combination that makes most sense to me while still being acceptable to the rest of the non-autistic world. Sometimes this is like trying to spell the word CAT from the letters A and T. The subsequent choices of combinations actually as witnessed gives me no clue as to the answer that I must come up with. I search my mind for possibilities of that which is missing while looking for a sign of acceptance or rejection from the agitated players who are already impatient with me. If real experiences could be put together and looked up in a book that was similar to a dictionary of experiences, then I would understand, easier, each event that I experience as a complete and meaningful happening. Wally Wojtowicz, Jr. [253]

One of the ways to counteract the loss of the why questions is through the use of Social Stories. This method of communication with children with autism was developed by

Carol Gray at Jenison High School, in Jenison, Michigan. Books on how to develop and use social stories for children with autism are available through Future Horizons, Inc.[254] Some children react best to the story format, others to visual pictures where the story is sketched out, instead of written with words.

Conclusion

As a fitting finale for this chapter on social interaction I would like to share two statements by Thomas McKean.

> These children, despite what statistics say, DO have intelligence! They KNOW when they are being patronized, they KNOW when you are talking about them behind their back. Please, PLEASE treat them with respect and the dignity you would with anyone else. They deserve this. And I feel that you will also see some improvement. Those of you who work with the autistic population, please watch yourselves. Very few things hurt us as bad as others thinking we are aliens or babies. We are not. We are people. Flesh and blood with thoughts and feelings. Feelings which can be, and are, easily hurt.[255]
>
> Remember that somewhere inside each of them lies a real person. A person with thoughts and feelings, and a person who needs love just as you do. And if you do not give it to them, no one will.[256]

231 The American Psychiatric Association, *Diagnostic and Statistical Manual of Mental Disorders, Fourth Edition* (Washington, DC: American Psychiatric Association, 1994) pp. 70-71.

232 Lurline Morphett, *Face to Face* (Adelaide, South Australia: Publications Branch, Education Department of South Australia, 1986) p. 14.

233 Leo Kanner, "Autistic disturbances of affective contact," in *Classic Readings in Autism*, Anne Donnellan, ed. (New York: Teacher's press, 1985) p. 41.

234 Leo Kanner, p. 42.

235 Dietmar Zoller, *Wenn ich mit euch reden konnte...* (Bern, Germany: Scherz Verlag, 1989). Introduction translated by Annie Humphreys, Autism Research Unit, Sunderland Polytechnic, Sunderland, Great Britain.

236 "What is Autism Anyway?" *Alberta Heritage Foundation for Medical Research Newsletter*, (Edmonton: Alberta Government Publication: 1989).

237 Judy Barron and Sean Barron, *There's a Boy in Here* (New York: Simon and Schuster, 1992), p. 181.

238 Donna Williams, *Somebody Somewhere* (Toronto, Ontario: Doubleday Canada Limited, 1994) p. 95.

239 Thomas McKean, An Alternate Look at Autistic Perceptions [Cassette recording # 930713-580] (Richmond Hill, Ontario: Audio Archives of Canada, 1993).

240 Judy Barron and Sean Barron, pp. 138, 144 & 180.

241 Therese Jolliffe, Richard Lansdown and Clive Robinson, " Autism: a personal Account," *Communication* (Vol 26, no. 3, 1992) p. 13.

242 Therese Jolliffe, Richard Lansdown and Clive Robinson, p. 13.

243 J. Bemporad, "Adult recollections of a formerly autistic child," *Journal of Autism and Developmental Disorders* (Vol. 9, no. 2, 1979) p. 192.

244 J. Bemporad, p. 193.

245 Thomas McKean, "An inside look at auditory training," *The Advocate* (Vol. 25, no. 1, 1993) p. 14.

246 Mary McCracken, *A Circle of Children* (Philadelphia: J.B. Lippincott Co., 1973) p. 97.

247 Sharisa Kochmeister, "FC and the controversy surrounding it. The 'whens', 'whats', 'whys' and 'wishers' - a personal and objective informative view. How can we answer the questions if they won't listen? or If a tree falls in an empty forest, is there any sound at all?" *Living with the Questions* (a conference sponsored by The Facilitated Communication Institute and Syracuse University, May 21, 1996)

248 Therese Marie Ronan, personal correspondence.

249 Temple Grandin and Margaret Scariano, *Emergence: Labeled Autistic* (Novato, California: Arena Press, 1986) p. 69.

250 "What the DSM-IV means to me...", from the Internet, March 1996, address: http://www.udel.bkirby /asperger/asmeansl.html.

251 Sara Miller, "Does the Princess have PDD? Family gatherings" Autism Society of Southeastern Wisconsin Newsletter (November, 1993).

252 Sara Miller, "My personal autism spectrum theory" Does the Princess Have PDD? (unpublished manuscript, 1993). Used with permission.

253 Wally Wojtowicz, Jr., personal communication, permission granted to quote.

254 Books on Social Stories, by Carol Gray, include: *Original Social Stories, New Social Stories, Comic Strip Conversations, Taming the Recess Jungle,* all published by and available through Future Horizons, Inc. Arlington, TX. (800) 489-0727.

255 Thomas McKean, "An inside look at auditory training," p. 14.

256 Thomas McKean, "An alternate look at autistic perceptions," in *Proceedings from Autism: World of Options Conference* (Toronto: The Autism Society of America and Autism Society Canada, July, 1993).

Chapter Nine

Intelligence

The mother of a four-year-old child who has autism was worried. She was sending her boy to preschool and he could not even say his own name. In her anxiety, she asked her son "What is your name?" over and over again, hoping he would respond appropriately. Instead he answered clearly. "I'm not 'tupid, Mom."[257]

This child had been tested and found to be at a retarded level of development. He was also diagnosed autistic. Studies have clearly shown that sixty percent of all individuals with autism score below 50 on the standard IQ test.[258] Twenty percent of them score between 50 and 70. The remaining twenty percent score over 70. According to the DSM-IV "approximately 75% of children with Autistic Disorder function at a retarded level."[259] Obviously, this child was mentally incompetent and must be treated so. When doctors were questioned about his "I'm not 'tupid" quote, they replied, "he is only mimicking words someone else has told him."

A young man in Australia was observed using a new method of communication developed for nonverbal individuals.[260] Louis is twenty-four years old and attends an Adult Training Centre designed for people who are too disabled to be admitted to sheltered workshops. He speaks a few involuntary phrases that do not seem to make any sense.

After some work on a talking computer, Louis was introduced to the Canon Communicator, on which the instructor showed him the alphabet and numbers. Only thirty minutes after starting this whole process, Louis typed out his name on his own. Then, when asked if there was anything he wanted to say, he typed "IM NOT RETARDED" and "MY MOTHER FEELS IM STUPID BECAUSE I CANT USE MY VOICE PROPERLY." His next statement was a question, "HOW MUCH IS A CANNON?"

A mother in England was concerned about the care that her son, who has autism, was receiving in a state facility. He told her of various situations which were upsetting to him and could be easily dealt with by the staff. When she relayed this information to the staff members, they informed her that he was only manipulating her by telling her these things. They had no answers themselves on how to help this lad, so they chose to administer more drugs. He spent his days sitting on the floor, holding his teddy bear and rocking.[261]

A seventeen-year old with autism went for psychological testing. Although nonverbal, he apparently understood everything people said to him, and reacted accordingly. He was administered a vocabulary test. The first page went well. He pointed to the correct answer. The psychologist turned the page and the boy reacted. She was turning the pages backwards. He attempted to show her how to turn them forward. She did not comply and asked the next question. He refused to answer. She continued on for the next few pages, asking the questions. He was visibly upset every time the page was turned backwards and continued to refuse to point to any of the answers. She sighed and closed the book, marking him down at the vocabulary level of a two-year old child.

We questioned her on why a test for individuals with autism was designed backwards when it is common knowledge that those who have autism like to have things go in order. She replied that it makes it easier for the psychologist to administer the test. We argued that it was obviously no indicator of the lad's vocabulary level. She said it was all she could do. The results were entered in his medical records.

A teenager with autism took several different IQ tests in several different situations and with several different examiners. The test results varied from a low of 40 to a high of 160. Guess which results ended up in his permanent records?

A preschooler's IQ was tested with his mother watching through a one-way window. The child correctly answered every item on the test. The examiner began to ask the questions over again and the child was visibly confused. He looked at the examiner; he looked over all the answers intently and then hesitantly chose a different answer. This continued throughout all of the repeated questions. The mother asked the examiner why the questions were repeated? He replied that repeating the questions eliminates guesswork. The mother then asked, "Didn't you see the change in my child's behaviour? Couldn't you see that he understood that the repetition of the question meant that he had got it wrong in the first place? Couldn't you have explained to him what was going on?"

"No," was the reply, "any explanation would affect the results". Does this mean that the lack of an explanation has no effect on the outcome of the test? In IQ testing there is a big difference in getting 100% of the questions correct, and getting half of them wrong, especially when that half means that all answers are treated as guesswork. Another label of mental retardation has been unjustly applied.

It is time for parents, professionals, and educators to stand up and demand that children, clients, and students be treated with respect and fairness when it comes to intelligence testing. There is not a single intelligence test which has been normed for an autistic population, especially if sensory stimulation is taken into account.[262] The development of these tests assumes that they will only be used on the populations they have been normed for. By applying them to the autistic population and then using these scores as life-long labels, we do a grave injustice.

When Temple Grandin was a child, she was diagnosed by doctors as severely brain damaged.[263] Her parents were advised to put her away in an institution. Her mother refused to believe that she was a vegetable and ignored the medical opinion. She fought for speech therapy and a fair education. Today, Temple holds a Ph.D. in Animal Science and has a successful career as a designer and consultant to ranchers, meat packers and corral managers around the world. She has written a book on her experience as an individual with autism and travels extensively as an advocate for people with autism.

Dietmar Zoller is a man from Germany who has also shared his life experiences in two books: *Wenn ich mit euch reden konnte...* and *Ich gebe nicht auf.* Although Dietmar does not speak, he reads and writes German, English, and French. Again, it was his mother who refused to give in. After learning to read and write on his own, Dietmar realized that he was not stupid and developed a great hatred against people who treated him as if he was feeble minded.[264] Once, in a rage, he threw an apple at a teacher; a frustrated attempt to show what he thought of him without the use of words. Dietmar is now actively campaigning for greater understanding of people with autism in Germany and works as a translator for the German Autism Society.

David Eastham, a Canadian with autism, was given little hope of communicating by his teachers.[265] His mother taught him to read when he was fourteen using shaped letters and phonics. He went on to take college courses in which he got A's. He also wrote very moving poetry which has been published in the books *Understand* and *Silent Words*. He reveals an emotional sensitivity that is likely felt by all people with autism, but one which they are unable to express.

Parents of children who have autism want to do their best. They desperately search far and wide for answers that make sense. They go to professionals who claim to know what they are doing and find that labels are applied; labels that last a lifetime. Deep in their hearts the parents know the labels are wrong. They resist and try to speak out. Instead of listening to their concerns, many professionals reach into their black bags and pull out more labels. The parents are treated for denial.

As caregivers to this population, we must be aware of the lack of concrete evidence on the IQ levels of the autistic population. A lack of verbal communication makes almost every IQ test invalid. Methods of administering these tests bring grave doubts as to their ability to measure those who have autism accurately. Assumptions that those who have autism are mentally handicapped affects our response to them. As long as we assume that they are incapable of learning, we do little as educators.

Firmly entrenched in our society are numerous attitudes and beliefs which must be given up. Lack of verbal ability does not indicate mental retardation. Motor problems, lack of fine motor skills and/or a lack of coordination does not indicate mental retardation. Unacceptable, unpredictable and bizarre behaviours do not indicate mental retardation. Until we can let go of these concepts, people with autism will continue to have trouble reaching their full potential as we will be the ones standing in their way.

Individuals with Autism Say ...

> I wanted to live up to the potential of my brain, but I was confined to this body that seemed to have its circuits crossed or shorted out. I attended special education classes that were conducted on a preschool level. That meant that I had to do boring tasks such as stringing large wooden beads or placing pegs in a pegboard. Or I had to listen to a word spoken by the teacher and then point to a picture of the object.
>
> But I did learn to read. I taught myself. Mommy had a cassette tape of the alphabet, which she used to play for me over and over. I learned my letters. Then when I was watching television with the family, I would connect those letters with the ones I saw in commercials. Little by little I began to read words, then sentences. I even leaned over the back of Daddy's chair and read from his book or newspaper. Eventually I became a fast reader, able to recall a whole page after just a glance. Ian Wetherbee[266]
>
> Although my IQ tested at 130+, I was placed in the slower paced reading and math groups. What they didn't understand was that I was trying to learn, I just learned differently from other kids. Anything that was visual or logical, something I could draw or see, I could learn. I couldn't learn any other way. [267]
>
> i do want you to know what its like inside autistic children without touching on the writing we are lets say so scared its a fear like no other can you imagine what its like living in a social system that is always saying youre crazy it embodies such products of elementary evil that there is no way to describe it i want everyone to know that autistic children arent stupid the way people often think
>
> i can think clearly inside my head and i can feel too but when i want to put the so called simplest actions into breathtaking practice in these

> surroundings outside the crate I can't do it restlessness comes over me anxiety and idiotic panic bring me almost to despair. Birger Sellin [268]

Kiyo Katahara is a teacher in Japan who developed a method of teaching children with autism called Daily Life Therapy. Through work with thousands of autistic children since 1964, she has come to the conclusion that the lower-functioning individuals with autism have higher levels of intellectual ability which are not being used.[269] If educators do not assume that ability is present, they choose to concentrate on teaching basic life skills to those who have autism. These students have been robbed of the use of their intellect for life.

Facilitated Communication is a method of communication developed for work with nonverbal populations.[270] In Facilitated Communication, a therapist lightly touches the client's hand or arm as messages are typed out on a machine, or pointed to on a communication board. There is a great deal of controversy about the actual source of the messages that are being communicated. Is the therapist creating the message, or is it actually coming from the individual with autism?

A large portion of the criticism is in relation to the content of the messages themselves. Supposedly retarded individuals are not only able to understand questions, but they are able to type out the responses, using words, feelings, and even spellings which do not fit our expectations. When asked where they learned how to read and to spell they come up with such avenues as cereal boxes, signs, and Sesame Street.[271] Self-taught in their silent worlds, those who have autism may actually realize far more of what is going on than most of us admit.

Extensive study has gone into the area of teaching normal students based on the individual learning style of each student. These styles are based on the idea that every person uses a preferential sensory system to process and store information.[272] Incoming information is represented by the visual, auditory, or kinaesthetic (touch) cognitive systems. Individuals usually have a primary system, but also may incorporate all three systems while learning. If we do not take into consideration the problems of sensory over stimulation in the autistic population, it is obvious we will not comprehend learning problems or solutions for those who have autism. We must realize that those who have autism need to learn how to use their specific senses in environments that are safe. We must also realize that the individual with autism will likely prefer to use the sensory system which is causing them the least trauma. For example, Temple Grandin says:

> I learned visually. The only thing I remember from math class was a hands-on demonstration on the meaning of "pi" - the formula for finding the area of a circle. I remember that the teacher took a cardboard circle and wrapped a string around the circumference and showed the class that it equalled three diameters with a little left over which worked out to 3.14. This was real to me. I saw it and understood it.[273]

For students like Temple Grandin and Sara Miller, visual aids are extremely important for understanding. However, other individuals who have the greatest area of difficulty with their eyes will likely respond better to auditory or kinaesthetic learning methods. One woman learned most successfully through the use of touch.[274] She learned how to put her shoes on the right feet by running her finger along the side of her foot and the sides of the shoes.

As educators, we must realize that it is as imperative to assess the individual cognitive learning style of students with autism as it is with any one else who is having learning difficulties. It is also imperative to realize the importance of providing safe sensory stimulation if we expect to be able to teach these children anything.

We must also be aware that those who have autism may have abilities which are far beyond our own. A young child who is able to count automatically as a whole may never benefit from someone teaching him how to count one by one. If you can toss a dozen items on a table and the child instantly responds with twelve as the amount, is it really necessary to force him to count each item up to twelve? Obviously this child has a talent. Is it not better to attempt to work with this talent and see how far it can be developed rather than force our inferior methods of counting on him, driving him to boredom?

Another child can play classical music on the piano by ear and automatically transposes it into another key when he so chooses. He may do this to avoid using a key on the piano which is slightly out of tune. To insist that he play only the simple pieces the teacher chooses as appropriate for his age level, and in the "proper" key means that we will likely turn off his interest in playing the piano for a lifetime.

The ability to learn to read is a major concern for parents with children who have autism. Often parents report that their children are reading very early in life -- such as at two years of age. Other children are fascinated with books and spend hours sitting and turning the pages. These children are usually considered to bc using the books as obsessions, with little thought of them actually reading. Why? Because the books they choose are for adults, with small printing and no pictures. The assumption that it is impossible for children to learn to read on their own at such an early age or that they would choose to read adult literature sets limits on children that will affect any of our efforts to school them. Dietmar Zoller[275] and Birger Sellin[276] are two examples of children who taught themselves to read long before anyone even realized their intellectual potential.

Another reality we must deal with when working with individuals with autism is boredom. This can be apparent in both areas of learning and testing. If we assume the student is incapable of learning we will only provide the simplest of materials. If we are unable to test the student's acquisition of the material presented, we likely will assume it has not been learned and keep on teaching it. The student is never exposed to anything new.

I worked with one young man who went through twelve years of schooling at a kindergarten level. As a common technique of the education system of the era, he was kept in a separate classroom for children with learning difficulties. Each year attempts were made to teach him colours and shapes, how to count, the alphabet, and other simple tasks. The rest of his time in the classroom was spent putting together jigsaw puzzles. Twelve years of his life were wasted in this manner. Integration with peers is eliminating such horror stories in some schools, but unless teachers are aware that those who have autism are capable of learning, they will not take the responsibility to find ways in which children with autism can utilize the information.

Supplying an education, which is both interesting and relevant to the student, is also important. The following is an excerpt from a letter a young man wrote to one of his teachers:

> Hello Alex. I do speak to you indirectly through the written words because I can not explain by speaking to you in person.
>
> I think you asked me what I wanted to learn at school and you was always trying to discuss things with me to decide what I was to decide to do.

I have told you that I want to learn physics, chemistry, mathematics, artists.

Why will you not respect my wishes and listen to my opinion.

I want to know these subjects. How would you feel if you did choose to learn and people frustrated you.

Paediatricians said that I was retarded not intelligent but you thought that I was clever and I decided that you were my extra special friend.

I am intelligent you should have asked appropriate questions for college students as we are just equally as capable of learning.

I was happy with you because you tried decisions to help me make. A friend dear which I knew.

You Alex treated me with respect as a friend.

Richard[277]

Repetition of information is one of the fastest ways to develop boredom for students. As Sara Miller points out "I only had to hear or read it once and I remembered. I didn't need it repeated a thousand times!"[278] When Temple Grandin looked back at her school years she realized that her misbehaviour in school was directly linked to boredom and the thrill of wondering what would happen if she were caught.[279]

Testing can also lead to boredom, and thus become meaningless. Thomas McKean describes his experiences as a young child being dragged from one professional to another as his parents looked for clues to his odd behaviour. He says that it didn't take long for the tests, which were repeated over and over again, to become boring.[280] There is only a small amount of satisfaction in putting the round peg in the round hole. For him, testing became a means of trying to invent new and different ways to solve the problems.

Obsessions

Obsessive interest in a single topic or object is a common problem in the area of autism. Individuals become obsessively interested in one subject to the point that they block out everything else. This may happen for a number of reasons, the first and foremost is likely the need for protection and the desire to control the environment in order to provide that protection. This reaction is best illustrated throughout the book *There's a Boy in Here* by Judy and Sean Barron.[281] Other obsessions may indicate an aptitude for one subject such as math and the feeling of success when one takes part in it. Still others may be an extreme example of the individual interests everyone develops as a human being. I expect my son has as much understanding of the joy and fascination I get from my collection of elephants, than I do of his comic book and memorabilia collection. Accepting these interests and differences in interests is far more important than an exact understanding. We do it for normal people; why are we so reluctant when it comes to people who are disabled?

Teachers, who are trying to instil a certain amount of knowledge in their students, may well feel that they have come up against a wall when they hit the obsessive interests of a student with autism. Two choices can be made. One can concentrate on eliminating or ignoring the obsession or one can use the obsession by directing it into constructive channels in the areas one is teaching. A good example of this type of teaching was carried out with

Temple Grandin, who was obsessed with cattle chutes.[282] Her teacher used her interest in this area to motivate an interest in science. His understanding led her to a career in the design of livestock handling systems.

Other fascinations in Temple Grandin's past were not accepted by her teachers. An obsession with election material in elementary school may well have been used to stimulate interest in social studies, history, government, geography and math. Instead teachers and psychologists focused on elimination of the obsession. A wonderful opportunity for learning was lost for good.[283]

Coming up with creative ways to use the obsessions of a student with autism is a challenge well worth facing. By using the interests of the child to motivate learning, as teachers, parents and other caregivers, we have the opportunity to build rather than destroy.

Imagination

Experts claim that people with autism do not experience fantasy, or use their imaginations. This is not supported by individuals with autism who are speaking out or by the majority of parents who know their children well. Neither is it supported by observable behaviours.

A mother talks of her twin sons using fly swatters for sword play after they had seen a movie on television.

One child created a game of pool from an assortment of balls and sticks after watching a movie in which dogs played billiards. He played this game on the steps by himself, and with anyone else who wanted to join in.

Another child was observed lying in a window seat at his father's house talking about Carol, a neighbourhood baby. He began acting as a baby and did not stop when his Dad and I joined in by treating him like a little baby. This episode concluded with this child crawling up into his father's arms, curling up like an infant and pretending to suck on a bottle, all the time making appropriate baby noises.

These are only a few examples of imaginative play I have observed or have had reported to me. In order to understand the lack of imagination in an individual with autism's world, we must not forget the main focus of life for those who have autism. They are in a situation in which protection from pain is of prime importance. Imaginative play usually is forsaken for the need to protect and control the environment. However, when a safe environment is provided, the child is free to use imagination in any way he chooses.

We may be blind to what is actually going on in the mind of the person with autism. Their choice of play behaviour may not fit our expectations. That doesn't mean it is any less imaginative to them.

> Friends have never been stimulating or entertaining enough for me. When I was younger, I lived in a world that was heavily layered. I was usually watching myself and my activities through a third party. Not unlike a camera watching an actor pretending to be someone else's life. I was very inflexible and needed to do things my way. It was too difficult to explain to friends what I was doing and I was never interested in doing things the way they wanted to. I had a great imagination - maybe too good. I was always busy in some elaborate fantasy - so it was difficult to break out of that and play with dolls or some other type of role-playing with other kids.

Another problem with playing with other kids is that they weren't as interested in the same things I was. For awhile I was obsessed with being a crossing guard. Later, my fascination turned into getting hurt. Neither of these things are conducive to other children playing with me. I would pretend that I had something cut, sprained or broken. I would make slings and crutches with anything I could find. I had one set of crutches made from tent stakes and croquet mallet heads. Curtain rods were another thing to use as canes or crutches. I'm certain that I was a great embarrassment to my parents and neighbours. I didn't really care and when I actually did get hurt, the attention scared me to death.

Today I enjoy working on my computers, swimming, playing computer or Nintendo games. I no longer have any interest in getting hurt or being a crossing guard.[284]

The need for protection often intensifies the fears of those who have autism as they use their imaginations to deal with their day-to-day lives. Antisocial behaviours of peer groups are often exaggerated as a danger to the individual.[285] The howl of the wind can be transformed into a typhoon, a cyclone or a flood by an overactive imagination.[286] The combination of acute sensitivity and the constant need for protection does not allow them much freedom to use imagination for pleasure. Once they are given the chance to live in environments that are safe from over stimulation, and thus pain, they are also given the chance to be free to use their imaginations and they will do so.

Method of Care

Never assume retardation. Some individuals with autism work better in the morning than the evening due to biochemical build up in their systems. It may prove beneficial to concentrate on educational activity in the mornings. Concrete methods of teaching seem to work far better than the use of abstract ideas. Use as many visual techniques as possible to pique interest.

Be well prepared to fill the day with activity. People with autism have difficulty filling in the empty spaces of time until they have been taught how to do so.

The environment and sensory problems must always be taken into account in any form of instruction for a student with autism. Otherwise we are just wasting our time and theirs, much like trying to teach a blind person to read in the normal fashion. This does not mean that they have to be removed from normal environments; it just means that we have to be aware of the problem, and deal with it when necessary.

The environment and sensory problems must also be taken into account whenever tests are administered.

Obsessional interests can be used to stimulate interest in the various subjects taught in school and to motivate reading, research, exploration, and, most of all, learning.

Physical education should be part of any good education program. Problems with noise and tactile contact mean that students with autism will not enjoy, or desire to take part in, team sports.[287] These environmental factors cause the problem, not the fact that people with autism cannot be competitive, which is so often assumed. Consideration of these feelings should always be taken into account when planning the physical education program. Individual sports activities are preferable to team sports. A few examples of suitable sports are cross-country running, swimming, downhill and cross-country skiing, gymnastics, biking, skating, and weight training. A daily exercise program using callisthenics, aerobics, or the new step exercises may also be helpful, especially when one remembers to keep the music and instruction levels low.

Physical exercise produces good endorphins throughout our bodies which help us to cope with stress and anxiety. This is also true for the autistic population. Due to their heightened reaction to anxiety, physical exercise should be an integral part of every school day. The increased level of endorphins will lead directly to a more efficient level of concentration for learning tasks. Sara Miller believes that the lack of what she calls "fits" in school during her adolescent years was directly related to the one and a half hours of swimming she put in every morning as a competitive swimmer.[288] Sara finds that the twenty to thirty minute programs suggested for typical people are not sufficient as an exercise regimen. She needs at least an hour to an hour and a half to get the excess energy out of her system.

Trust is an all important factor in the education process, especially with those who have autism who are so sensitive to feeling. All children can feel whether or not we have faith in their abilities. If we do not believe in those with autism, they will not cooperate. They also will not make any attempt to communicate with us. The frustration of having to deal with our negative attitude leads to higher levels of agitation and unacceptable behaviours.

> When the teacher is well prepared and assumes all students are capable, I sit quietly and behave. When the teacher is disorganized and assumes we are stupid, I can't control my outbursts. Awful feelings come over me and I have to leave the classroom. Sue Rubin[289]

> All my life I was enrolled in classes for the profoundly retarded. The pain of that isolation, I can't describe. Some classes consisted of putting flashlights together and then they would be taken apart for the next days project. I never spoke or made eye contact. I hummed and self-stimmed. No wonder they thought I was hopeless. I was always treated well but my intellectual needs were never addressed because nobody knew I had any intellect at all. Sad to say, many like me remain in that same hellish situation. Dan Treacy[290]

Once the attitudinal and environmental factors are in place, we may be able to teach individuals with autism much like we do any other student. Personally, I favour the use of imitation, much as I did with my own children when they were young. Teachers have their own individual method which works the best. Feel free to use it!

We must also be aware that the younger the child is when exposed to this method, the swifter and more beneficial the results will be. Because of historical factors, older individuals may have greater obstacles to overcome. A person develops over time. The older we are, the more resistant we are to change. However, never be afraid to try. Finding a reason for one's differences can affect those who have autism in ways we cannot predict.

In the book *A Circle of Children*, teacher Mary MacCracken describes her work at a school for emotionally disturbed children, many of whom have autism. Although she does not recognize the sensory problems these children have, she does realize the importance of accepting the unique individual character of each student and going from there. Effective teaching must include a deep sense of caring for each student so that one gets to know each personally and take their differences into account.[291] For children with autism, the importance of accepting them personally may well be as important as working with their heightened sensitivities.

Conclusion

Although studies have shown that the majority of the autistic population is retarded, I do not feel that I have ever met an individual with autism who is actually retarded. On the other hand, I have met many who have not developed their capabilities, due to the environments and situations in which they have been raised. They may live in what appears to be a state of retardation. Their need for protection has taken precedence over learning information and acquiring abilities related to certain tasks. Until we take this factor into account, society will continue to believe that they are mentally retarded and treat them as such.

This, of course, does not mean that there are not any individuals with autism who are also mentally retarded. It means I just haven't met any of them, yet. However, I am certain that the number with mental retardation is much lower than the 75% cited in the DSM-IV. It is likely more closely related to the percentage of so-called normal individuals who suffer from mental retardation.

Measuring a nonverbal child in an educational situation is very difficult. Unless they pass certain tests they are often kept at a kindergarten level of education for most of their school lives. How can we expect them to learn, when all we expose them to is this limited amount of information year after year? If a lack of an appropriate method of communication stands in the way of passing tests, is it not more profitable to err on the side of too much rather than too little exposure to information? Instead of repeating grades, I believe it would be much more useful to move the child through the school system with his same age peers, allowing exposure to new information, even if we cannot measure what knowledge he has already acquired. In the meantime, we must also work on developing reliable methods to measure their abilities.

The assumption that these children are intelligent, not retarded; supersensitive, not disabled, need to learn to cope rather than be fixed, opens new doors of possibility for them. Let's turn their hopeless futures into ones filled with hope.

Every so often, I come into contact with the writings of people with autism that fill me with such awe that I wonder what I am trying to do, speaking out for these people who are so much more talented than I am. This is especially true of the published works of Temple Grandin and Donna Williams. Throughout my travels I meet other writers who have yet to be published. One of these writers is Wally Wojtowicz, Jr., a young man from the state of New York.

Wally sent me a collection of his writings after I met him in Syracuse, NY in May 1996. As I go through them, the lessons we can learn about those who have autism, are numerous. However, they are also written in such a wise and compelling manner, one does not have the heart to shorten or take excerpts from them. Instead, I feel they should be published in their entirety, which does not fit well into the scope of this book. However, I feel that Wally's comments on the long-term effects of his treatment in the classroom are a lesson that each of us should not miss out on. Therefore, I am including this article.

As a young man, Wally recently had the opportunity to attend a presentation on autism and education. Speakers at the workshop included Temple Grandin, as well as a panel of speakers from a school that Wally attended as a child. This answer was written by Wally in response to a question from his father. The name of the school and teacher have been changed with Wally's permission. I have also taken the liberty of dividing it into more paragraphs in order to make it easier to read.

As you read through this article, remember that the person who wrote this has been considered mentally retarded and incapable of understanding his own feelings, much less those of other people. His need for protection from stimulation from the environment means that he is almost constantly involved in using repetitive behaviours to block out our world. It is a fine example of how wrong we can be when we depend on appearance to define any person. I hope it also gives each of you the motivation to look closely at those with whom you are living and working on a daily basis. Perhaps they too understand our world far better than we dream possible.

"Wally, let's talk about the meeting that you went to today. What did you think of the information, as presented, for the professionals and students to learn from?"

> In opinions this forces me to talk frankly, freely and light-heartedly, rest assured. I thought the delivery of our food should have been faster. It was slower, typically, than I like. Gaylan, you know, is looking good for her age. You are slowly looking better too.
>
> The meeting, as an informational function for teachers, professional and popular folks, was too boring to make me get excited because I am not as interested in school procedural philosophies and functions in the community as I am in the functioning attitudes of the teachers, administrators and other staff as pertaining to their association with their students and the community. The panellists from Green Lake School did a fine job for the students, so in that sense it was, Pop, worth while. Temple's presentation gave hope to those who say that opportunities for the autistics don't exist.
>
> The best and most interesting part of the function for me was Temple's presentation. Grandin's direct and unusual style pleases those in the audience. It is mostly opinion on my part that I find her more refreshing each time I listen to her.
>
> Temple, if judged for her beauty, would probably not win the prize. In time, people will displace their bigoted opinions about her outward appearances, social roughness, and inability to develop eye contact with her audience, and instead, see a lovely human being right before their eyes. Temple is to be, Pop, finally recognized through her books, engineering and her opinions about firm pressure to relieve nervous tension and for her contributions to the understanding of the autistic mind. In general, I give her high marks for the meeting.
>
> It is through this type of public education that the hypocrisy held by some segments of the society towards the handicapped is dispelled. Human frailties, or human greatness, when viewed in the same mirror, are merely reflection of the same things, too. They reflect the mind of the person looking humbly back at you. Those discernible and recognizable subtle human differences, together, establish the boundaries that effectively delineate what we steadfastly consider to be the social backbone of our social hierarchical system.
>
> We tend to place good looking, smooth talking individuals in the upper echelons of our social scale. These are what we call beautiful people. At the

opposite end of the scale are the handicapped, forced to hide there in their shadowy existence and be subjected to gross intolerance by people at a slightly higher level and above. In between these extremes we sense as white and black, are those people who reside in what is known as the grey scale with its thousands of shades of human imperfection, which are benignly overlooked and tolerated.

Often, by structuring our society in this way we are giving up that which is good, true, and sometimes great for that which is erroneous or nice or fiction. We are like insects being attracted to a bright light or sweet smell, even if these are bait for a disaster. This is typical, Pop, of our society's continuing quest for the truth.

I give Temple the greatest respect that I look for from others. Grandin is the inspiration for me to do the things that I dream of. Grandin is the articular of a segment of the population having no voice or identity, but having, intact, a mind and will to fight on up to greatness. Truth differs from fiction in that truth will find too many detractors in the present: fiction, as a substitute remains unchallenged in the present but cannot withstand the test of time. Grandin is giving those who relegate genius to only the normal population a jolt that should have been delivered a decade before.

Often, after time has passed, foolish notions about something or someone finally begin to fade. Dim light is to finding a needle in a haystack as time is to memories. I, however, remember very well the treatment I received at the hands of Mrs. Bezor. She represents for me the treatment that I received in all the programs I was in before I learned to communicate. Hopelessly, I kept trying to cooperate in the best ways that I could in all of the various programs. However, the finger bending punishment that I received in some programs just got continually worse, forcing me to endure bodily harm that I feel in my joints even today.

Her philosophy at that time was great for intimidating those children who could not understand their own language let alone understand a foreign accent which was superimposed on some variation of the Queen's English. Illusions of this torture passed through my mind as I listened to her speak. Segments of what she said somehow freed my mind, not of disdain for her, but of great amounts of guilt that I have been harbouring for years since I attended Green Lake School.

I prefer, for reasons of not wanting to remember the pain and humiliation I felt at that time, to not answer the question of why I feel guilty. I hope you realize that for sometime in my younger years during the time I was at Green Lake School, I experienced voices in my mind telling me very much as Mrs. Bezor did of how awful I was, especially, since I performed so terribly during school. The voices that I heard in my mind were those of dear Mrs. Bezor and a second unknown voice which added, too, lyrics of the refrain which played over and over in my mind.

I can remember fully the words that added the effects of despair, fear, danger, and worthlessness to my opinions about myself and my future. You are awful, retarded, a poor learner, dumb, disabled and destructive are some of the words and phrases that would flow through my consciousness, deepening the great chasm that would separate me from light and freedom and leave me alone to desperately try to escape a seemingly sterile and dark desert island. Her voice and ghostly figure would play the songs that I feared to taunt and torment me when she would not be physically present. She faded away once I was free of Green Lake School.

I didn't determine the details of these feelings which returned as I listened to Mrs. Bezor speak, but remembered the fear that I felt sometimes from just being in her presence. Dread, foreboding, anxiety and sheer terror are simply given over to mistrust and withdrawal in a young and confused mind. I find, now, that illusions immortalized in my mind by fear, withstood the test of time. In time, I you know, will find immortality through my writings and along with me, too, those people, who by either design or ignorance, sent me deeper into the hopelessness of my life, and too, those who were dear to me and educated me, hopeful trying to somehow deliver me from the darkness that kept me from freedom in my life.

Often, joyous and great memories are abruptly destroyed when tears of reality stream from my mind and pour out what is left of dignity and self worth over the edge of that which I am trying to frantically escape. In your eyes, Pop, I run just like everyone else, jump like everyone else, even look like everyone else, but in giving me this equality, you don't see the real me. The person you see is just a ripple, daring to be seen. A darting, small faceless, determined and assertive shadow of the deep and seldomly understood human being who is effortlessly gliding silently along the treacherous jagged edge of two worlds, while pensively and deliberately sipping frequently the sweet and fragrant nectar thought to hold the joys of life from both kingdoms.

It is without a doubt that I have learned from these reconnoiterings to either side of my desert, where the darkness is the only dimension that is not boundless. Nor is it totally discernible to warn of the occasional interloper of its sweet minglings of joy and ugly pain that we learn to accept as reality. That reality illuminates not my festering fruitless mind, but teases open, gradually, my intellect, appreciation of life, intense desire to fill just one life with love, appreciation of God, and finding eternal the sense of peace and joy that is longed for, universally, by all people.

Very rarely, if ever, can I find it bright enough in the light of reason and understanding to equate the frequently sinister offerings of gifts of help, understanding, trust and loyalty to those of joy, peace, friendship, love, better life, and kindness when I greatly distrust the bearer of the gifts. I always trust other autistics like Temple Grandin and Jim Sinclair because they share with me the uncorrupted definitions of love, peace, friendship, humility and kindness that represent the basics of our pure, simple and occasionally, naive visions of life and human relationships. In contrast, to trust another person whose response to these same values is qualitatively eroded by the additional pressures that frequently force a person to go against those values that nurtured their entire being detracts from their credibility thus hindering their reputation. Too many times, the values and principles of a person are so highly compromised that I cannot trust in their sincerity and as a result, I refuse to have a meaningful relationship with them.

Sincerity, represented by exaggerated kindness and concern from those people is easily recognized as being false. Each relationship grows in understated terms and is filled again and again with hope. In your heart is where you find the peace that trusting another person established itself and it resides hidden beneath the very feelings you find so valuable in others.

Dim sensations of fear followed by copious feelings of resentment begin to grow inside of yourself as you hear segments of the speaker's presentation fluctuate from what was to what is now politically correct. You wonder about the true motivation of the speaker's presentation and hope that, for now, instead of opportunities for her self-edification and advancement, she truly believes in that which she publicly espoused earlier at the meeting.

As I listened to her speak, I remembered thoughts that I had remembered during my time at Green Lake School. These thoughts and feelings were earlier experienced by me during my toddler years. As I look back, often looking for that which attributed to my autistic condition, I find that each experience I had involving intuitive sensations of mistrust, immediate disaster, or foreboding, was linked in some way to a person or to a place that frightened me or caused me harm of immense proportion either physically or psychologically. In this fear was borne yet another cause for my autism: my inability to trust people, even my own family.

Trust is looking to another person for what he or she does openly and without malice for another person for no particular reason other than kindness and love. In but a small number of instances did I experience this humanity operating at a discernible level: these involved my family and a few family friends and rarely involved the professional staff that I was in contact with. This inability to trust others, possible, was the greatest impediment to my psychological development that I am aware of. In retrospect, these early experiences of mistrust and incredible fear had guided me toward the blackness of fright and toward the great feeling of despair that knowing that I understood everything that I was exposed to but couldn't outwardly express brought on. The same feelings that I experienced as a toddler ran through my mind as I listened to the folks from Green Lake School give their glorious accounts of hope, kindness, friendship, devotion and caring that are the cornerstones of their programs as found at present. And soulfully wondered why it took them so long to realize that young children are looking for help and understanding, not ridicule, humiliation and regimentation.

Uppermost in my mind is the direction that the treatment of autistic children is headed. Opinions frequently detected in the tone and tenor of the presentations are what influences the audience's perception of the content of that which is presented and remembered by them.

Temple Grandin's presentation at this meeting will most certainly be remembered due to the fact that most people at the assembly still assumed that autistics were incapable of doing anything more than sitting in a corner and twirling a piece of string for hours on end. Her contribution to destroying those ideas is, perhaps, her greatest and most outstanding achievement. Together with Temple, the impact of the presentations of the two mothers of autistic boys, illuminated the minds of most of those present and gave real life and local affirmation to many of Temple's suggestions and ideas.

The professional staff from Green Lake showed the students and other attendees that, often, realignment in group thinking is necessary and is frequently brought about by new ideas and new theories about educating a segment of the population once thought to be doomed. Adding together what was presented at this meeting was the beginnings of a new paradigm in the education of autistic persons.

Perhaps educators of the handicapped will now be more inclined to realize that they should look at finding answers to the often asked question, "Is it worth the time and money to educate the handicapped child?" From opportunities like this meeting presented, I look at opportunities like these as opportunities for those early educators to hear themselves speak the words and listen to what they mean in light of what they have done in the past and in light of what they look for in the future, not from their students but from themselves. This meant as much to the Green Lake Group as it meant to the students of the local college and others present at the meeting.

Educators, together with those wanting to be educated should feel secure in knowing that we can both learn from each other if we keep open minds and establish a respectful relationship with each other, something that was totally missing during most of the time that I have been involved in special education programs. In conclusion I politely and delicately point out that educational opportunities for the front line staff are as important to the success of a program's outcome as is the education of the administrative staff. The program's success is the total effort of all who are involved and depends on the training and education of everyone, including the lunch room staff. END. Wallace Wojtowicz, Jr.

257 Gail Gillingham, "I'm not 'tupid, Mom," *Edmonton Autism Society Update* (Vol. 6, no. 4, December, 1990) p. 28.

258 Fact Sheet on Autism (Washington: United States Department of Health and Human Services, 1980).

259 The American Psychiatric Association, *Diagnostic and Statistical Manual of Mental Disorders, Fourth Edition* (Washington, DC: American Psychiatric Association, 1994) p. 67.

260 Douglas Bilken, "Communication unbound: autism and praxis," *Harvard Educational Review* (Vol. 60, no. 3, 1990) pp. 295-296.

261 Personal Correspondence from a mother of a son affected by autism.

262 Dr. Beth Fouse, *Creating a Win-Win IEP for Students with Autism* (Arlington, TX: Future Horizons, Inc., 1996) p. 37.

263 Rena LeBlanc, "Dustin Hoffman only played the part but I lived it," *Woman's World* (September 12, 1989) p. 10.

264 Dietmar Zoller, *Wenn ich mit euch reden konnte...* (Bern, Germany: Scherz Verlag, 1989). Introduction translated by Annie Humphreys, Autism Research Unit, Sunderland Polytechnic, Sunderland, Great Britain.

265 Margaret Eastham, Silent *Words, a Biography* (Ottawa, Oliver Pate, 1992) p. 35.

266 Ian Wetherbee, "M-Y...N-A-M-E...I-S...I-A-N", *Guideposts, a Practical Guide to Successful Living* (August, 1993) pp. 4-5.

267 "What the DSM-IV means to me...", from the Internet, March 1996, (address: http://www.udel.edu/bkirby/asperger/asmeansl.html) p.2.

268 Birger Sellin, *I don't want to be inside me anymore* (New York: Basic Books, 1995) pp. 57 & 138.

269 Kiyo Katahara, *Daily Life Therapy A Method of Educating Autistic Children* Volume 1 (Boston: The Nimrod Press, 1983) p. 128.

270 Douglas Bilken, p. 291-292.

271 Paul Nichols (producer) Lisa Hsai (director), "Free from silence," *Prime Time Live* (New York: ABC, 1992).

272 Lloyd Flaro, *Mending Broken Children* (Edmonton: Learning Strategies Group Inc., 1989) p. 38-39.

273 Temple Grandin and Margaret Scariano, *Emergence: Labeled Autistic* (Novato, California: Arena Press, 1986) p. 60.

274 Therese Jolliffe, Richard Lansdown and Clive Robinson, "Autism: a personal Account," *Communication* (Vol 26, no. 3, 1992) p. 18.

275 Dietmar Zoller, Introduction.

276 Birger Sellin, p. 23.

277 Stella Carlton, *The Other Side of Autism* (Worcester: The Self Publishing Association Ltd., 1993) p. 143.

278 Sara Miller, "Does the Princess have PDD? Different is good: it's back-to-school time," *Autism Society of Southeastern Wisconsin Newsletter* (September, 1993).

279 Temple Grandin and Margaret Scariano, p. 60.

280 Thomas McKean, An Alternate Look at Autistic Perceptions [Cassett recording # 930713-580] (Richmond Hill, Ontario: Audio Archives of Canada, 1993).

281 Judy Barron and Sean Barron, *There's a Boy in Here* (New York: Simon and Schuster, 1992) p. 120.

282 Temple Grandin and Margaret Scariano, pp. 103-104.

283 Temple Grandin, "Teaching tips from a recovered autistic, " Focus on Autistic Behavior (Vol. 3., no. 1, 1988) pp. 5-6.

284 "What the DSM-IV means to me...", from the Internet, (March, 1996, address: http://www.udel.edu/bkirby/asperger/asmeansl.html) p. 3 & 5

285 Judy Barron and Sean Barron, p. 113.

286 Annabel Stehli, *The Sound of a Miracle* (New York: Doubleday, 1991) p. 171.

287 Sara Miller, "Does the Princess have PDD? What can you do with someone who is so sensitive?" *Autism Society of Southeastern Wisconsin Newsletter* (March, 1993).

288 Ibid.

289 Sue Rubin, "Killing Autism is a Constant Battle", *The Communicator*, newsletter of the Autism National Committee (Vol. 7, no.1, Spring 1996) p. 12.

290 Dan Treacy, "A Meditation", *The Communicator*, newsletter of the Autism National Committee, (Vol.7, no.1, Spring, 1996) p. 8.

291 Mary McCracken, *A Circle of Children* (Philadelphia: J.B. Lippincott Co., 1973) pp. 215-217.

Chapter Ten

Other Therapies

Auditory Training

Auditory Training is sweeping the world as a treatment for people with autism. This procedure was developed by a French physician, Dr. Guy Berard, to counteract the effects of deafness[292] and is based on the theory of exercising the ear through the use of different frequencies of sound. Auditory Training has had some excellent success stories, the most well known outlined in the book *The Sound of a Miracle* by Annabel Stehli.[293] Since the publication of this book, Dr. Berard has trained specialists from around the world. Other specialists are springing up, using their own treatment methods. Treatment takes ten days. This treatment works extremely well for some people with autism and has little effect on others.[294] Still others have reported an improvement in their hearing which disappears over time.[295]

I believe one has to look at the source of the procedure and the sensory abilities of the person we are working with to understand just why and when this method works. Auditory Training was developed to correct damage to the ears.[296] It is obvious that people with super-sensitive hearing may well have received damage during their lives. Therefore, one would expect the most success with this treatment with people who have the greatest level of difficulty with hearing. Little or no improvement will be found with those autistic individuals who suffer more in the area of tactile or visual sensitivity.

As we have mentioned earlier, sensitization occurs when a person reacts so strongly to a response it results in a higher level of reaction to similar stimuli in the future.[297] High acuity to sound may well lead those who have autism to a constant state of sensitization if they are exposed to sounds which cause trauma. Auditory Training may well be the procedure which allows people to return to their normal state of hearing. Their hearing will still be acute, but the response will no longer be as strong.

Auditory Training may be beneficial to any individual with autism, especially those who have problems with sound. I would suggest that parents look into this therapy. Be prepared to have little or no improvement and to pay a relatively high cost. Be cautious as to where and how specialists in this area are trained and exactly which method they are using.

Another therapy linked to Auditory Training is called the Tomatis Method.[298] This also uses frequencies to repair damage to the ears. Tomatis is based on the idea that the mother of the autistic child did not connect with the child when in the womb and that the child has to relive this experience by hearing the sounds an infant hears before it is born.[299] Tomatis therapy takes much longer than Berard's Auditory Training and costs quite a bit more. As with Auditory Training, there are reports of success and failure with this therapy.[300]

Facilitated Communication

Facilitated Communication is another therapy that is receiving a great deal of attention at this time,[301] and one which is also steeped in controversy. Facilitated Communication does not offer any hope of a cure, but instead gives the nonverbal individual the opportunity to communicate. Facilitated Communication was developed by Rosemary Crossley in Melbourne, Australia. It was brought to the United States by Douglas Biklen of Syracuse University after he visited Australia to study the methods. It challenged all his beliefs about autism. He was convinced that Facilitated Communication worked and through his efforts, its use has spread throughout the United States and Canada and is being used in schools, group homes, institutions and homes.

Facilitated Communication allows a nonverbal person to speak by using a letter board, keyboard, typewriter or computer. A facilitator lightly touches the hand or arm of the person communicating, which gives that person the freedom to type out a message. Controversy is based primarily on the source of the message relayed - by the facilitator, or the autistic person - as well as other factors which have been presented in other areas of this book.[302] Much of the negative reaction to FC stems from the lack of response when the disabled person is not touched and incorrect responses when the facilitator is unaware of the correct answer. Testing this method of communication has also proved almost impossible as the individuals do not respond well in a test situation. However, some parents, teachers and caregivers who have been exposed to this method of communication are extremely positive about its usefulness.

One of the biggest benefits of this therapy is the voice provided for more autistic people. If we listen, as caregivers, we have the chance to understand. Empathy, through understanding, can only lead to better care in the long term.

Messages received through Facilitated Communication have strengthened the argument of sensory over stimulation as a major factor in autism.[303] As more research is done in this area, and more people take the time to try and understand the actual feelings and experiences of individuals with autism, we should see more information developing on specific ways to help them.

If you are working with a nonverbal autistic individual, I would not hesitate to recommend the use of Facilitated Communication. However, I would also suggest that one also speak very softly and keep the environment as quiet as possible. If we can give them the chance to speak on their own, we are providing a greater gift. The use of letter boards, typewriters and computers can also make a big difference in the lives of people who are tactile sensitive and cannot stand holding a pen or pencil to write. The more methods we can access for communication, the better off we all are.

As facilitators, we must be extremely conscientious that we are not, in fact, producing the messages that are being communicated. If there is any question in our own minds, we must admit that we may have a problem. Using individuals with autism to convey our own words - even unintentionally - robs them of the faculty of communication and may well lead to an insistence in society that this method of communication be discarded for this population.

In order to understand how Facilitated Communication works with sensitive individuals, one has to look at the use of human touch with people who are upset. A woman, presented with a medal for her volunteer work, is overcome with emotion as she tries to say thanks. The light touch of a friend's hand on her arm calms her enough to continue her speech. Human touch is calming to each of us.[304] Light human touch can and does calm the autistic individual. By lowering the stress level of those who have autism, we give them the ability to carry out tasks that are usually too much for them to deal with. As the person becomes used to communicating - a very stressful experience for someone who has not done it before - the touch of the facilitator can become lighter and lighter. In time, some individuals learn to communicate without anyone touching them.

One of the unique problems that has developed through the use of Facilitated Communication has been allegations of sexual abuse.[305] In the past two years, more than 20 formal sexual abuse charges have been made in the United States, based solely on information garnered through Facilitated Communication. Until Facilitated Communication can be validated by scientific means, these charges are likely to go nowhere.

I believe this issue is also one in which we, as caregivers, must be very cautious to not use assumptions based on our own attitudes and beliefs to judge what the person with autism may actually be telling us. The horrifying reality of sexual abuse is finally being taken seriously throughout the world, but we may be too quick to jump on that bandwagon instead of really listening to what the autistic individual is telling us. Free at last, to open themselves up to the world, they may well be sharing feelings of over stimulation we do not take for granted.

For example, I once dealt with a four-year old foster child who had been taken from her father due to neglect, stayed with a close friend of mine for a time and finally moved into the home of a foster mother who specialized in the care of disabled children. She had recently taken courses which focused on recognizing the signs of sexual abuse. One of the signs of abuse was the lack of desire or willingness to be touched by anyone. Like many other persons with autism, this young girl demonstrated this behaviour. Based on this sign the foster mother insisted that the girl had been sexually abused in the past by her father, and that the child needed treatment for this abuse, although there was nothing in her previous records to substantiate this claim. The foster mother would not listen to anyone who tried to tell her that the withdrawal from physical contact may well be a feature of her autism, not of sexual abuse.

When individuals with autism are describing problems of their past, especially in tactile areas and stating that certain people hurt them, we must be aware that any touch is painful and that they are not necessarily speaking about sexual encounters. We must be extremely cautious about jumping to any conclusions in this area, or adding our assumptions to what is being communicated to us. On the other hand, those who have autism are as vulnerable to sexual abuse as anyone else. They have the right to be respectfully listened to and protected from this crime. Make absolutely certain you are not affecting the communication you are facilitating.

Sensory Integration

Sensory integration was developed by physical therapists in the United States and Canada.[306] It has become a popular therapy in many areas of developmental disability with reports of positive results. Debra Cook has developed a specialized program using sensory integration with students with autism in the classroom.[307]

The focus on sensory stimulation might lead one to believe that this therapy would fit well within the method of care outlined in this book. Be aware that there may be differences, especially in the attitudes of the therapists. For some, sensory integration may be based on the theory that the sensory response system of the individual is dysfunctional and needs to be fixed rather than giving the person the opportunity to learn to cope with his or her individual abilities. Therapy may also concentrate on producing "normal" behaviour patterns, which may well do more harm than good as outlined in the visual chapter. Eliminating certain behaviours or responses is definitely questionable unless one has considered the whys and hows of the behaviour carefully. For example, looking straight ahead at a task may be preferable to teachers and other caregivers who want a normal response. On the other hand, if the vision is blurred and the task is thus more difficult, one would wonder why being "normal" is so important.

Sensory integration can be an excellent addition to this whole method of care if the actual feelings and experiences of the individuals are taken into consideration. One must realize that bombardment with stimulation, which is often part of these programs, may lead to the person reaching the point of shut down and thus feeling better for a period of time after therapy. On the other hand, the bombardment may just provide higher levels of over stimulation which will cause additional stress and anxiety to the individual with autism. They will then have to retreat further into themselves for protection. Be aware that many of the sensory integration suggestions are effective as they act as replacements for the repetitive and stereotypic behaviours used by those with autism.

All in all, I believe that sensory integration is well worth investigating. Many of these methods of therapy can be easily incorporated into a program which considers the environment and over stimulation. Other methods may provide an opportunity for the autistic individual to desensitize parts of the body so that they are no longer painful when used. An example might be the desensitization of the finger tips so that working with pencils, zippers and eating utensils is possible.[308]

Holding Therapy

Holding therapy was developed by Martha Welch[309] and is another method of treatment which ties directly back to the theory of refrigerator parenting. Today, it is rejected by most people in this area of care.

Holding therapy is based on the premise that children with autism did not receive adequate comfort as infants from their parents, and therefore need extra holding now. During this therapy the child is held very tightly by one or both of the parents, who talk calmly and lovingly throughout the therapy. Watching this exercise can be heartrending as the children become more and more agitated and fight the restraining arms of their loving parents. Finally the child reaches a breaking point and submits. Exhausted, they may accept the love of their parents and sometimes even offer their own.

As we consider the information shared in this book it is easy to understand what is going on through the holding process. In fact, holding is even suggested as a method to restrain very agitated individuals. However, there is a big difference between creating agitation for your children and helping him deal with his own agitation. Yes, holding therapy appears to work. Yes, the child might become more open and normal after bouts of holding therapy. The question we must ask is - "Are the long term results worth the trauma and stress we are forcing the child to endure?" A woman who has experienced this form of therapy describes it as terrible suffering which achieved nothing.[310] She attributes the submission of the children as an act of exhaustion. Temple Grandin responds to holding therapy with this philosophy: there are two ways to train a horse, through gentleness and through force. Both training methods may well do the job; which in the long run is better?[311]

Behaviour Modification

Behaviour modification is the method of therapy most widely used with the autistic population at this time and which is most often suggested in autism pamphlets as a treatment method. The main force behind behaviour modification comes from California, led by Dr. O. Ivar Lovaas.[312]

Behaviour modification is based on the elimination of undesirable behaviour by the use of rewards and the shaping of desirable behaviours. The problem with this method of treatment is that it is directly concerned with specific behaviour, paying no attention to the reasons behind the behaviour. As we have discovered, the bizarre behaviours have a reason. These behaviours are used for protection, and until the protection is provided the individual must cope in some way. Sure, certain behaviours may well be eliminated during behaviour modification, but others will only take their place.

Behaviour modification is disturbing to me as it indicates that there is only one "normal" way of reacting to the world and that each and every one of us must follow that pattern, no matter the circumstance. Throughout the years, this method of treatment has reported a high level of success. However, in the long run, many people with whom it has been used as the main focus of treatment are unable to lead unsupervised adult lives.[313] They now spend their lives in group homes and sheltered workshops.

The term behaviour modification has now been replaced by Applied Behaviour Analysis (ABA). It is recommended as an early intervention treatment for children with autism by many people. Be cautious of any program that does not take the sensory sensitivity of those with autism into account.

Vitamins and Minerals

The main crusader for the use of vitamins and minerals as a treatment for autism is Dr. Bernard Rimland[314] at the Autism Research Institute in San Diego, California, but research in this area has been done throughout the world and shows positive results.[315]

Vitamin therapy is based mainly on administration of Vitamin B6 and the mineral magnesium. Vitamin B6 is important to our bodies as it normalizes metabolism.[316] The results of this change in metabolism are normalized brain waves and urine chemistry as well as improved behaviour. Magnesium is required in the body to utilize the Vitamin B6.[317] Therefore, a combination of these two supplements are required in any treatment program of this type.

Several studies have been carried out with different amounts of vitamin B6 and magnesium being administered daily, over different time periods. Studies done by Dr. Rimland reported global or partial improvement in a majority of the subjects.[318] Most studies also reported a deterioration in behaviour when the treatment was discontinued.

Dr. Rimland proposes that a megavitamin formula is more beneficial than just a vitamin B6 and magnesium treatment and suggests a product that contains a multitude of vitamins and minerals as well as the suggested amount of 500 mg of Vitamin B6 and the 250 mg of magnesium per teaspoon.[319] He suggests that parents try this supplement for up to ninety days. If no improvement is recognized by that time, it is safe to conclude that this child does not require extra B6.[320]

The only parents to whom I have talked and are using the vitamin therapy with their children are also combining it with specialized diets based on suspected allergies. The response of these parents to the combined therapy is very positive. Videos taken before treatment and again after several years of treatment also indicate a significant improvement.[321]

Diet

Diet Therapy for an individual with autism may be based on diets developed for hyperactive children and consist of removing all sugar, food dyes, milk products or substances that have been determined to cause an allergic reaction to that specific individual.[322] As far as I can find, there are few scientific studies that focus on these diets and the effect they have on autistic behaviour. Other diets are based on the problem of candida or yeast infection in an individual.[323] These plans remove all yeast products and sugars from the diet. An antifungal medication may be administered as part of the program. Again, improvements are based on anecdotal information rather than actual scientific studies.

However, diets based on the total removal of casein and gluten have been developed and significant improvement in the autistic condition has been reported.[324] These diets are based on the abnormal patterns found in 24-hour urine samples of the subjects. The patterns indicate an insufficient breakdown of the proteins gluten (which comes from wheat, rye, barley and oat) and casein (which is found in milk products.)[325] It is believed that a direct result of the incomplete breakdown is the increased level of certain peptides in the body. These peptides affect the brain chemistry directly and inhibit the breakdown of other peptides.

Fifteen children with autism have followed a gluten and casein free diet in Norway for several years. Changes in behaviour for all 15 children were documented in the first year: they became easier to work with, less resistant to learning, and developed an increased concentration span.[326] There was a decrease in the level of fear, bizarre movements such as flapping and a change in sensory reaction. For example, one young lad was pleased to be able to wear a bandage on a cut. In the past he could not stand the sensation of having a bandage on his skin. After four years, continued improvements are reported, especially in the areas of linguistics and cognitive abilities, or the ability to both understand and use the information received.[327]

The researchers do not claim that this diet is a cure for autism, but a method to allow the children to become more attentive and receptive and thus able to make use of the education they are receiving.[328] I believe that work in this area is extremely important as it ties directly to the biochemical make-up of the brain and the differences found in the autistic population. These differences may well explain the super sensitivity of those who have autism and produce new methods to cope with it.

Daily Life Therapy/Seikatsu Ryouhou

Daily life therapy was developed as a method of education for children with autism by Dr. Kiyo Kitahara in Japan.[329] This program is currently being carried out at the Higashi schools in Tokyo and Boston.

Daily life therapy is based on three main features.[330] The first is the need for emotional stability based on high self-esteem and a pursuit of independent living. Secondly, the method focuses on improved physical strength, which is achieved through a thorough program of physical exercise. Regular patterns of eating and sleeping are also stressed. The third focus is the stimulation of the intellect through instruction in all areas of language, arts, mathematics and social sciences. Instruction is based on the individual ability of each child, as well as their interests. The therapy works from a premise that children with autism have the potential to be normal and thus need a well-rounded education. Expression is encouraged through the use of art and music. Group activities are used for the development of communication and social skills.

At present, Daily Life Therapy is only available to the students of the Higashi Schools. Costs are high. Research is being carried out in Boston as to the efficacy of the methods used by the Higashi School. Information from this study may be useful in the development of more effective educational programs for children with autism. As with most programs in the field of autism, I can find little mention of the sensitivity to sensory stimulation in any of the reports on Daily Life Therapy. However, a sensitivity to emotional feeling is definitely recognized.[331, 332]

Option Method

The Option Method of therapy for autism was developed by Barry and Suzi Kauffman of the United States and is based directly on the Option philosophy.[333] Although I have read the book *Son Rise*, which describes using this therapy during the early years of their autistic son's life, I have had little time to delve further into this method. Therefore, I will summarize a report from an observational program conducted by Rita Jordan of the United Kingdom in 1990.[334]

The Family Program at the Options Institute in Massachusetts does not claim to effect changes in the individual child, but focuses on training the family to work with the child and to train other volunteers in this method once the family returns home. The Method is quite expensive and requires that parents learn it at the Massachusetts centre.

The key ideas of the Option approach are that our behaviours are determined by our understanding of the situation, and what is best for us at that time; that we can learn to recognize and challenge our underlying beliefs and always have a choice or an option. Finally, choosing to be happy in a situation means we accept it, that we love people as they are, rather than as we would wish them to be.

In this method of care for the child with autism, acceptance is the key issue. However, as far as I can find, little or no recognition is given to the state of super sensitivity to sensory stimulation in individuals with autism. A particular sensitivity to the "real" attitudes of people who are working with them is assumed, based on the way children with autism react to others. Sensitivity to touch, sound, sight, smell, and taste, as well as to emotion, is ignored. Therefore, the Option Method does not fit well with the scope of our book.

However, since acceptance of the autistic situation is a particular focus of this method, the Option program may give people the opportunity to learn how to accept others. In fact, parents and professionals I have talked to, who have been involved in the program, or who have dealt with people who have been involved, claim that the Option Method does much more for the parents and other family members than it does for the child with autism. Learning to accept that we have a choice to be happy or unhappy with a particular situation is a very important lesson.

Conclusion

The above therapies, although only a small sampling of the many available were included because they seem to have the most followers and thus the greatest effect on our autistic population.

Therapies stressed in the past, such as psychotherapy or the use of electrical shock, are no longer accepted by the majority of the psychological or educational communities as being useful or ethical. However, it is wise to be aware that many professionals who are not actively involved in the field of autism at this time may well have been taught that these individual methods of treatment are not only acceptable, but the only treatments available. For example, the main treatment focus for autism in the French community is psychotherapy, based on the refrigerator parenting theory. When we are dealing with professionals who get most of their information from publications which are written in French, we will likely discover a firm belief that psychotherapy is the only answer to autism.

Many people may never have to deal with autism during their careers. Thankfully, most people working in this area are open and actively involved in learning as much as they can in order to work effectively with their clients.

Another treatment with which to be cautious is the use of drugs. Medical practitioners who have little knowledge of autism are often very willing to prescribe one type of psychotic drug after another in an attempt to deal with the problems caused by this syndrome. I claim no expertise in this area, but remind parents and other caregivers to be very cautious when it comes to the administration of any drugs to those who have autism. Epilepsy or some form of seizure activity is often a real factor in the life of a person with autism and medication may be necessary to control the seizures. Some adults with autism have discovered that low levels of anti-anxiety drugs bring enough relief to allow them to function more effectively in their daily lives.[335]

Peter Begin, an American psychiatrist, is very vocal about the lack of information on the long term effects of use of most psychotic drugs.[336] He also speaks to the lack of information psychiatrists share when negative effects have been discovered, with not only those they are treating but also with their caregivers. For some reason, the attitude that one need not inform seems to increase when one is dealing with a syndrome, such as autism, in which people are nonverbal and considered mentally incompetent.

292 Guy Berard (Keynote Speaker), "Auditory Training," [Cassette Recording No. 930713-410] 1993 International Conference on Autism, A World of Options (Richmond Hill, Ontario: Audio Archives International, Inc., July, 1993).

293 Annabel Stehli, *The Sound of a Miracle* (New York: Doubleday, 1991) p. 156-158 and 165-169.

294 Annabel Stehli, p. 200.

295 Thomas McKean, "An inside look at auditory training," *The Advocate* (Vol. 25, no. 1, 1993) p. 14.

296 Guy Berard, Cassette Recording No. 930713-410.

297 Stephen Kosslyn and Olivier Koenig, *Wet Mind The New Cognitive Neuroscience* (New York: The Free Press, 1992) pp. 384-385.

298 Timothy Gilmor, "Overview of the Tomatis Method" (Paper presented at the Ontario Psychological Association Annual Meeting, February, 1982).

299 Timothy Gilmor, p. 4.

300 John Kershner, Richard Cummings, Kenneth Clarke, Audrey Hadfield and Barabra Kershner, "Two-year evaluation of the Tomatis Listening Training Program with learning disabled children," *Learning Disabled Quarterly* (Vol. 13, Winter, 1990) pp.50-51.

301 Douglas Bilken, "Communication unbound: autism and praxis," *Harvard Educational Review* (Vol. 60, no. 3, 1990) pp. 295-296.

302 Stephen Calculator (Moderator), Tony Attwood, Richard Simpson, Brenda Smith Myles, Mary Knostantareas, Greg Gravelle and John Palmer (Panel), "Keynote Panel: Facilitated Communication," [Cassette Recording No. 930713-250] 1993 International Conference on Autism, A World of Options (Richmond Hill, Ontario: Audio Archives International, Inc., July, 1993).

303 Paul Nichols (producer) Lisa Hsai (director), "Free from silence," Prime Time Live (New York: ABC, 1992).

304 Ashley Montagu, Touching The Human Significance of the Skin Third Edition (New York: Harper & Row, Publishers, 1986) p. 46.

305 Richard Saltus, "Don't Touch Me," *The Edmonton Journal* (Sunday, July 18, 1993) p. F6.

306 A.J. Ayres, *Sensory Integration and the Child* (Los Angeles: Western Psychological Corporation).

307 Debra Galvin Cook, "A sensory approach to the treatment and management of children with autism," *Focus on Autistic Behavior* (Vol. 5, no. 6, 1990) pp. 1-19.

308 For more information on sensory integration, contact Sensory Integration International, 1402 Cravens Avenue, Torrence, California, 90501.

309 Martha Welch, "Appendix I: retrieval from autism through mother-child holding therapy," in *Autistic Children New Hope for a Cure*, N. Tinbergen and E.A. Tinbergen, eds. (London: George Allen & Unwin, 1983) pp. 322-334.

310 Therese Joliffe, Richard Lansdown and Clive Robertson, "Autism: a personal account," *Communication* (Vol. 26, no. 3, December, 1992) p. 16.

311 Temple Grandin, "An autistic person's view of holding therapy," *Communication* (Vol. 23, no. 3, December, 1989) p. 76.

312 O. Ivar Lovaas, *The Autistic Child Language Development Through Behavior Modification* (New York: Irvington Publishers, Inc. 1977).

313 Winnie Settle, "Impact innovative model program for autistic children and their teachers," *Edmonton Autism Society Update* (Vol. 7, no. 2, June 1991) p. 19.

314 Bernard Rimland, Enoch Callaway, and Pierre Dreyfus, "The effect of high doses of vitamin B6 on autistic children: a double-blind crossover study," *American Journal of Psychiatry* (Vol. 135, no. 4, 1978).

315 J. Martineau, B. Garreau, C. Barthelmay, E. Callaway, and G. Lelord, "Effects of vitamin B6 on average evolved potentials in infantile autism," *Biological Psychiatry* (Vol. 16, no. 7, 1981) pp. 635-636.

316 Bernard Rimland, Form letter regarding high dosage vitamin B6 and magnesium therapy for autism and related disorders, publication # 39D (San Diego, California: Autism Research Institute, 1989).

317 Bernard Rimland, 1989, p. 1.

318 Bernard Rimland, 1989, p. 1.

319 Bernard Rimland, 1989, p. 3.

320 Bernard Rimland, 1989, p. 2.

321 Bernard Rimland, 1989, p. 5.

322 More information on this therapy is available from Dr. Bernard Rimland, Autism Research Institute, 4182 Adams Avenue, San Diego, California, 92116.

323 William Crook and Laura Stevens, *Solving the Problem of Your Hard-to-Raise Child* (New York: Random House, 1987) pp. 282-287.

324 William Crook and Laura Stevens, pp. 285-287.

325 Ann-Mari Knivsberg, Kristi Wiig, Gunnar Lind, Magne Nodland and Karl Reichelt, "Dietary intervention in autistic syndromes." *Brain Dysfunction* (Vol. 3, 1190) p. 315.

326 Ann-Mari Knivsberg et al., p. 316.

327 Ann-Mari Knivsberg et al., pp. 323-325.

328 Ann-Mari Knivsberg, Magnus Nodland and Karl Reichelt, "Gluten and/or casein free diets as treatment," in *Proceedings from the Therapeutic Approaches to Autism: Research and Practice Conference* (Durham: Autism Research Unit and The National Autism Society of Great Britain, 1991) p. 165.

329 Kiyo Kitahara, *Daily Life Therapy A Method of Educating Autistic Children* Volume 1 (Boston: The Nimrod Press, 1983).

330 Paul Hardy and Daniel Edwards, "The efficacy of daily life therapy at the Boston Higashi School," in in *Proceedings from the Therapeutic Approaches to Autism: Research and Practice Conference* (Durham: Autism Research Unit and The National Autism Society of Great Britain, 1991) p. 116.

331 Kiyo Kitahara, Volume 1, p. xiv.

332 For more information on this subject there are three volumes of *Daily Life Therapy A Method of Educating Autistic Children* written by Kiyo Kitahara.

333 Barry Kaufman, *Son Rise* (New York: Warner Books, 1976).

334 Rita Jordan, "Two conflicting therapies?: the Option Method and Behaviorism as treatments for the fundamental difficulties of autism," in *Proceedings from the Therapeutic Approaches to Autism: Research and Practice Conference* (Durham: Autism Research Unit and The National Autism Society of Great Britain, 1991) pp. 91-98.

335 Temple Grandin and Margaret Scariano, *Emergence: Labeled Autistic* (Novato, California: Arena Press, 1986) p.141.

336 Peter Breggin, *Psychiatric Drugs, Hazards to the Brain* (New York: Springer, 1983).

Chapter Eleven

Returning to the Source

In the preface to the book, *Autism: Nature, Diagnosis and Treatment*, Geraldine Dawson shares this fable of Nasrudin.[337]

> A friend discovers Nasrudin on his knees, searching for his lost key. The friend joins in the search, and after a time, asks Nasrudin exactly where the key was dropped. He replies "In my own house." The friend then asks, "Why are you searching out here?" Nasrudin answers, "There is more light here than inside my own house."

The book's editor goes on to use "light" as a metaphor for the theories and technology of science and explains that light from a variety of sources is currently being used to discover a new understanding in the nature, diagnosis and treatment of autism. It has been four years since this book was published, and the autism field is still as confusing and frustrating as ever. New theories come and go. Methods of treatment become popular and then gradually fade away as something else becomes the new rage.

To date the "light" of science has not provided any real answers and even at the end of the century, the cause of autism is still unknown. There still is no cure. Much of the information available on this subject is filled with contradictions and discrepancies. Parents, teachers, caregivers and even the professionals continue to try to do their best with a limited amount of resources.

There is a chance this confusion will soon come to an end. Throughout the world people are turning away from the "light" and returning "home to look for the key where it was first lost." This movement started in an interesting field, not in research, but in entertainment. In 1989, the producers of the film *Rainman* first looked to actual individuals with autism to describe their experiences in our world. Since then, more and more individuals with autism are speaking out, and the professional world is gradually beginning to accept these descriptions as very important.

At the Los Angeles Conference on Autism in 1990, a panel of six adults with autism spoke at one of the sessions about their experiences. Additionally, one individual with autism was given one-third of a session to present her views. At the 1993 conference, four speakers with autism offered their own sessions, a panel of four other individuals with autism made up one session and in three other sessions, speakers focused on information gleaned directly from the autistic population. An obvious interest was indicated by conference participants as these sessions were all overcrowded and doors were either locked early, or sessions moved to larger rooms. Around the world, the "light" of science is being brought "into the house" as research projects based on these descriptions are beginning to take shape.

Throughout the world, the unique qualities of individuals with autism have been stressed to the point that caregivers are being forced to develop individual styles of treatment for each and every client. It is time to realize that people with autism also have many similarities. It is time to focus on how those who have autism are the same, rather than how they are different. The similarities are the basis for their autistic label. They also provide clues to effective methods of treatment.

Is acute sensitivity the cause of autism? If one looks to the *Diagnostic and Statistical Manual of Mental Disorders, Fourth Edition*, and particularly to Appendix A, for a description of the symptoms of autism, (see Chapter 1) one can definitely link each of these symptoms back to acute sensitivity. It may well be a cause. If one considers the similarities between the descriptions of individuals with autism, instead of concentrating on the many differences, one might again assume that it is a cause. To date, nothing else has made any sense.

If sensitivity is not the cause of autism, we still must take the time to recognize that it plays a very major role in the life of most, if not all, individuals with autism. Therefore, it is time that the professional community begin to concentrate on the role of super sensitivity in autism. By dealing with their sensory responses to the environment in a positive manner, we may give individuals with autism the chance to allow us access to more of their feelings and experiences.

Questions arise as to the source of the acute sensitivity. Is it, as I suggest, a physiological difference of a normal population sample which is linked to the genetic background of the individual? Or is it a biochemical dysfunction in the brain which can be discovered, monitored and perhaps manipulated to produce normality?

In order to answer these questions, the professional community must take the time to consider the reality of acute sensitivity in the world of the individual with autism, and measure not only the levels of sensitivity, but also the effects of these levels on the people involved. More research must be carried out on the various biochemicals in the brain and the effects they have in regards to sensitivity. The impact of diet and digestion on the production of these biochemicals must be measured. Differences in the womb and during the birth process should be measured in regards to sensitivity. The possible avenues for study are limitless, but will not begin take place until we listen.

This research will take years to accomplish. Until we have definitive answers, we must be willing to help those who have autism cope in the best way they are able. By following the program outlined in this book, as well as listening and trying to understand each individual we work with, we can provide a measure of hope.

If you, as caregivers, have personal doubts about the message in this book, I suggest that you share it with persons who have autism and watch their reaction. If they are able to read, allow them to read it and make up their own minds. If they cannot read, tell them what has been said and watch their response. If you are dealing with someone who is low-functioning, do this only when they are calm, relaxed, and not lost in a world of their own. Remember to speak very softly.

A father, who has known about this theory for several years and has cut down stimulation in his daughter's life, hesitated in sharing the information with her, just in case it might be wrong. He realized that sharing the knowledge was a big part of the method of care, but did not want to make that commitment. Finally, one evening he realized that he could not avoid it any longer and as he tucked his daughter into bed he began telling her about super sensitivity to stimulation. As he talked, he watched her physically change before his eyes. The tension she had lived with, all eight years of her life, flowed out of her body and has not returned.

If you are cautious about sharing this with individuals who are low-functioning because you do not think they can understand, you may want to try sharing the information with someone else while the individual with autism is within hearing range. I have done this in group homes with the staff while the clients listen in a nearby room. To date, I have yet to come across anyone with autism who does not react positively. I am fully willing to admit this may not mean there are people with autism who do not suffer problems with sensitivity to stimulation - only that I have yet to meet them.

I do realize that some of the professional community may not be willing to accept this theory and method of care. It not only challenges the definitions of autism which they have developed throughout the years, but also negates years of effort and research, which cannot be easily discarded. However, one must question - who are the most important people to consider? Is it the professionals who have made mistakes in the focus of their life's work, or the people with autism who must live with the consequences of that misplaced focus?

I also realize there are many who will look at this book and claim that it is far too simplistic in nature. How can anything so simple have taken so long to discover? How can anything so simple work effectively? The reality of changing one's beliefs and attitudes is never that simple. The reality of working from the point of empathy and understanding is much more difficult than trying to normalize someone else to your own position. Simplicity enters the picture when we realize that the method actually works. Allowing those who have autism their own unique humanity is the key that opens the lock to the autism puzzle.

I feel it is of prime importance to be willing to be open and accepting to what people with autism are saying. They are the ones who are actually experiencing the effects of this condition and thus they know far more than any of the rest of us. Let us give them our respect by really listening.

337 Geraldine Dawson, *Autism: Nature Diagnosis and Treatment* (New York: The Guilford Press, 1989) p. xv.

Suggested Reading List (Updated)

Autobiographies

Barron, J. & Barron, S. (1992). *There's a Boy in Here*. New York: Simon and Schuster.

Blackman, Lucy (1999). *Lucy's Story: Autism and other Adventures.* Brisbane, Australia: Book in Hand.

Eastham, D.W. (1985). *Understand.* Ottawa: Oliver Pate.

Eastham, M. (1992). *Silent Words - A Biography The Story of David Eastham.* Ottawa: Oliver Pate. (Also contains the poetry of David: *Forever Friends.*)

Gerland, Gunilla (1996). *A Real Person.* Translated by Joan Tate. London: Souvenir Press.

Gerland, Gunilla (2000). *Finding out about Asperger's Syndrome, High-Functioning Autism and PDD.* London: Jessica Kingsley Publishers.

Grandin, T. (1995). *Thinking in Pictures and Other Reports from my Life with Autism.* New York: Doubleday.

Grandin, T. & Scariano, M. (1986). *Emergence: Labeled Autistic.* Novato, CA: Arena Press.

Hale, Mary Jane Gray and Hale, Charles Martel Jr. (1999). *"I had no means to shout."* Bloomington, IN: 1st Books Library.

Lawson, Wendy (1998). *Life Behind Glass: A Personal Account of Autism Spectrum Disorder.* Lismore, Australia: Southern Cross University Press.

Lawson, Wendy (2001). *Understanding and Working with the Spectrum of Autism: An Insider's View.* London: Jessica Kingsley Publishers.

Martin, R. (1994). *Out of Silence -- A Journey into Language*. New York: Henry Holt & Co. (Actually written by an uncle but has some nice quotes from a child with autism; more difficult to read as it is a study of human language).

McDonnell, Jane Taylor and Paul (1993). *News from the Border: a Mother's Memoir of her Autistic Son.* New York: Ticknor and Fields. Note: the afterward of the book is written by Paul.

McKean, Thomas. (1996). *Light on the Horizon*. Arlington, TX: Future Horizons, Inc.

McKean, Thomas. (1994). *Soon Will Come the Light*. Arlington, TX: Future Horizons, Inc.

Miedziak, David (1993). *My Autobiography.* Autism Society of North Carolina.

Morphett, L. (1986). *Face to Face*. Adelaide, South Australia: The Publications Branch, Education Department of South Australia.

O'Neill, Jasmine Lee (1998). *Through the Eyes of Aliens: A Book About Autistic People.* London: Jessica Kingsley Publishers.

Reed, Dan (1996). *Paid for the Privilege: Hearing the Voices of Autism.* Madison, WI: DRI Press. Note: although the author does not have autism, there are many direct quotes from people who do.

Schneider, Edgar (1999). *Discovering my Autism: Apologia Pro Vita Sua (with apologies to Cardinal Newman).* London: Jessica Kingsley Publishers.

Sellin, Birger (1995). *I Don't Want to be Inside Me Anymore -- Messages from an Autistic Mind.* New York: Basic Books.

Shore, Stephen (2000). *Beyond the Wall: Personal Experiences with Autism and Asperger's Syndrome.* Shawnee Mission, KS: Autism Asperger Publishing Co.

White, B.B. & White, M.S. (1987). Autism from the inside. *Medical Hypothesis*, 24, 223-229.

Willey, Liane Holliday (1999). *Pretending to be Normal.* London: Jessica Kingsley Publishers

Willey, Liane Holliday (2001). *Asperger Syndrome in the Family: Redefining Normal.* London: Jessica Kingsley Publishers.

Williams, Donna (1998). *Autism and Sensing: The Unlost Instinct.* London: Jessica Kingsley Publishers.

Williams, Donna (1996). *Autism: An Inside-out Approach.* London: Jessica Kingsley Publishers.

Williams, Donna (1996). *Like Colour to the Blind.* New York: Times Books (a division of Random House).

Williams, Donna (1995). *Not Just Anything.* Arlington, TX: Future Horizons, Inc.

Williams, Donna (1994). *Somebody Somewhere Breaking Free from the World of Autism.* Toronto: Doubleday Canada Limited.

Williams, Donna (1992). *Nobody Nowhere The Extraordinary Autobiography of an Autistic.* Toronto: Doubleday Canada Limited.

Zoller, D. (1989). *Wenn ich mit euch reden konnte...* Bern, Germany: Scherz Verlag.

Zoller, D. (1992). *Ich gebe nicht auf.* Bern, Germany: Scherz Verlag.

Parent and Family Accounts

Christopher, W. & Christopher, B. (1990). *Mixed Blessings.* Arlington, TX: Future Horizons, Inc.

Copeland, J. (1976). *For the Love of Ann (Based on a Diary by Jack Hodges).* London: Severn House Publishers.

Fling, Echo (2000). *Eating an Artichoke: A Mother's Perspective on Asperger's Syndrome.* London: Jessica Kingsley Publishers.

Gerlach, Elizabeth (1999). *Just this Side of Normal: Glimpses in life with autism.* Eugene, Oregon: Four Leaf Press.

Gilpin, R. W. (1993). *Laughing and Loving with Autism.* Arlington, TX: Future Horizons, Inc.

Gilpin, R. W. (1994). *Move Laughing and Loving with Autism.* Arlington, TX: Future Horizons, Inc.

Gorman, J. (1997). *The Seeing Glass.* New York: Riverhead Books

Greenfeld, J. (1978). *A Place for Noah.* San Diego, CA: Harcourt Brace Jovanovich, Publishers.

Greenfeld, J. (1986). *A Client Called Noah.* San Diego, CA: Harcourt Brace Jovanovich, Publishers.

Hart, C. (1994). *Without Reason.* Arlington, TX: Future Horizons, Inc.

Hundley, J. (1971). *The Small Outsider, The Story of an Autistic Child.* Sydney, Australia: Halstead Press.

Junker, K. (1964). *The Child in the Glass Ball.* (G. Lannestock, trans.) Nashville, TN: Abingdon Press.

Kephart, B. (1998). *A Slant of Sun.* New York: W.W. Norton & Company,

Kaufman, B.N. (1976). *Son Rise.* New York: Warner Books.

Lovell, A. (1978). *In a Summer Garment: The Experience of an Autistic Child.* London: Secker and Warburg.

Mialaret, Gerard J. (1996). *Dancing with Dragons: An Entire Family's Insights into a Disability.* Arlington, TX: Future Horizons, Inc.

Park, Clara Clairborne (1982). *The Siege: the first 8 Years of an Autistic Child with an Epilogue Fifteen Years Later.* New York: Little Brown and Company.

Park, Clara Clairborne (2001). *Exiting Nirvana: A Daughter's Life with Autism.* Boston, MA: Little, Brown and Company.

Rankin, Kate (2000). *Growing up Severely Autistic: They call me Gabriel.* London: Jessica Kingsley Publishers.

Renning, A. (1995). *The Ultimate Treasure Hunt.* Ann Arbor, MI: J.A.M.A.

Robinson, Wendy (1999). *The Gentle Giant.* London: Element Books.

Stehli, A. (1991). *The Sound of a Miracle A Child's Triumph Over Autism.* New York: Doubleday

Stehli, A. (Editor, 1995). *Dancing in the Rain -- Stories of Exceptional Progress by Parents of Children with Special Needs.* West Port, CT: Georgiana Org., Inc.

History of Autism

Bettelheim, B. (1976). *The Empty Fortress Infantile Autism and the Birth of Self.* New York: The Free Press. (This book was the best seller of the 1960's which proclaimed the theory of cold parenting and negatively affected the lives of so many of the adults with autism we are dealing with today.)

Dawson, G. (Ed.) (1989). *Autism: Nature Diagnosis and Treatment.* New York: The Guilford Press.

Delacato, C.H. (1974). *The Ultimate Stranger: The Autistic Child.* Novato, CA: Academic Therapy Publications. (The first book which focusses on the differences in the sesnory sensitivity of those with autism.)

Donnellan, A.M. (Ed.) (1985). *Classic Readings in Autism.* New York: Teachers College Press. (Contains a copy of the first paper published on autism, by Dr. Leo Kanner.)

Siegel, B. (1996). *The World of the Autistic Child.* New York: Oxford University Press. (A very good outline of the view of autism by the medical community in the 1990's. Little reference to the actual experience of autism.)

Ratey, John J. (2001). *A User's Guide to the Brain: Perception, Attention and the Four Theatres of the Brain.* New York, NY: Pantheon Books. (Explains the experience of autism with what we now know about the brain.)

Education

Armstrong, T. (1987). *In Their Own Way Discovering and Encouraging Your Child's Personal Learning Style.* Los Angeles: Jeremy P. Tarcher, Inc.

Biklen, D. (1993). *Communication Unbound: How Facilitated Communication is Challenging Traditional Views of Autism and Ability/Disability.* New York: Teacher's College Press.

Flaro, L. (1989). *Mending Broken Children Cognitive Ability Patterning for Successful Learning.* Edmonton, Alberta: Learning Strategies Group Inc.

Gray, C. (Ed.) (1995). *Original Social Stories.* Arlington, TX: Future Horizons, Inc.

Gray, C. (1994). *Comic Strip Conversations.* Arlington, TX: Future Horizons, Inc.

Hodgdon, L. (1995). *Visual Strategies for Improving Communication.* Troy, MI: QuirkRoberts Publishing. (Available through Future Horizons, Inc.).

Kelly, K. and Ramundo, P. (1993). *You Mean I'm Not Lazy, Stupid or Crazy? A Self-Help Book for Adults with Attention Deficit Disorder.* New York: Simon and Schuster.

Kitahara, K. (1983). *Daily Life Therapy A Method of Educating Autistic Children* (Volume 1) (FitzGibbon, A.M., Trans.) Tokyo: Musashino Higashi Gakuen School.

Kitahara, K. (1984). *Daily Life Therapy A Method of Educating Autistic Children* (Volume 2 and Volume 3). Boston: The Nimrod Press.

MacCracken, M. (1973). *A Circle of Children.* Philadelphia & New York: J. B. Lippincott Company.

Rothenberg, M. (1987). *Children with Emerald Eyes Histories of Extraordinary Boys and Girls.* New York: E.P. Dutton.

St. John, P. (1991). *The Secret Language of the Dolphins.* New York: Summit Books.

Simons, J. & Oishi, S. (1987). *The Hidden Child The Linwood Method for Reaching the Autistic Child.* Kensington, Maryland: Woodbine House.

Sensory Issues, plus...

Anderson, E. & Emmons, P. (1996). *Unlocking the Mysteries of Sensory Dysfunction.* Arlington, TX: Future Horizons, Inc.

Ackerman, D. (1990). *A Natural History of the Senses.* New York: Random House.

Ayres, J. (1979). *Sensory Integration and the Autistic Child.* Los Angeles: Western Psychological Services.

Bolles, E.B. (1991). *A Second Way of Knowing The Riddle of Human Perception.* New York: Prentice Hall Press.

Bowlby, J. (1984). *Attachment and Loss: Volume 1 Attachment* (2nd ed.). Middlesex, England: Penguin Books.

Faber, A. and Mazlish, E. (1982). *How to Talk so Kids Will Listen and Listen so Kids Will Talk.* New York: Avon Books.

Hutt, S. J. & Hutt, C. (Eds.) *Behavior Studies in Psychiatry.* Oxford: Peragamon Press.

Kagan, J. (1994). *Galen's Prophecy Temperament in Human Nature.* New York: Basic Books.

Montagu, A. (1986). *Touching The Human Significance of the Skin* (3rd Ed.). New York: Harper & Row, Publishers. (Be cautious with the description of autism. It is based on the cold parenting theory.)

Films

Arnall, D. (Producer), & Webb, T. (Director). (1992). *A is for Autism* [film]. London: A Finetake Production for Channel 4.

Guber, Peters & Peters, J. (Producers) and Levison, B. (Director). (1989). *Rainman.* United Artists Film.